T0259201

Gastric Surgery

Guest Editor

GEORGE M. FUHRMAN, MD

SURGICAL CLINICS OF NORTH AMERICA

www.surgical.theclinics.com

Consulting Editor
RONALD F. MARTIN, MD

October 2011 • Volume 91 • Number 5

SAUNDERS an imprint of ELSEVIER, Inc.

W.B. SAUNDERS COMPANY
A Division of Elsevier Inc.
1600 John F. Kennedy Blvd., Suite 1800, Philadelphia, PA 19103-2899
http://www.surgical.theclinics.com

SURGICAL CLINICS OF NORTH AMERICA Volume 91, Number 5
October 2011 ISSN 0039–6109, ISBN-13: 978-1-4557-1155-0

Editor: John Vassallo, j.vassallo@elsevier.com
Developmental Editor: Teia Stone

© **2011 Elsevier Inc. All rights reserved.**

This journal and the individual contributions contained in it are protected under copyright by Elsevier, and the following terms and conditions apply to their use:

Photocopying
Single photocopies of single articles may be made for personal use as allowed by national copyright laws. Permission of the Publisher and payment of a fee is required for all other photocopying, including multiple or systematic copying, copying for advertising or promotional purposes, resale, and all forms of document delivery. Special rates are available for educational institutions that wish to make photocopies for non-profit educational classroom use. For information on how to seek permission visit www.elsevier.com/permissions or call: (+44) 1865 843830 (UK)/(+1) 215 239 3804 (USA).

Derivative Works
Subscribers may reproduce tables of contents or prepare lists of articles including abstracts for internal circulation within their institutions. Permission of the Publisher is required for resale or distribution outside the institution. Permission of the Publisher is required for all other derivative works, including compilations and translations (please consult www.elsevier.com/permissions).

Electronic Storage or Usage
Permission of the Publisher is required to store or use electronically any material contained in this journal, including any article or part of an article (please consult www.elsevier.com/permissions). Except as outlined above, no part of this publication may be reproduced, stored in a retrieval system or transmitted in any form or by any means, electronic, mechanical, photocopying, recording or otherwise, without prior written permission of the Publisher.

Notice
No responsibility is assumed by the Publisher for any injury and/or damage to persons or property as a matter of products liability, negligence or otherwise, or from any use or operation of any methods, products, instructions or ideas contained in the material herein. Because of rapid advances in the medical sciences, in particular, independent verification of diagnoses and drug dosages should be made.

Although all advertising material is expected to conform to ethical (medical) standards, inclusion in this publication does not constitute a guarantee or endorsement of the quality or value of such product or of the claims made of it by its manufacturer.

Surgical Clinics of North America (ISSN 0039–6109) is published bimonthly by Elsevier Inc., 360 Park Avenue South, New York, NY 10010-1710. Months of publication are February, April, June, August, October, and December. Business and Editorial Offices: 1600 John F. Kennedy Blvd., Suite 1800, Philadelphia, PA 19103-2899. Periodicals postage paid at New York, NY and additional mailing offices. Subscription prices are $311.00 per year for US individuals, $532.00 per year for US institutions, $152.00 per year for US students and residents, $381.00 per year for Canadian individuals, $661.00 per year for Canadian institutions, $429.00 for international individuals, $661.00 per year for international institutions and $210.00 per year for Canadian and foreign students/residents. To receive student/resident rate, orders must be accompanied by name of affiliated institution, date of term, and the *signature* of program/residency coordinator on institution letterhead. Orders will be billed at individual rate until proof of status is received. Foreign air speed delivery is included in all *Clinics* subscription prices. All prices are subject to change without notice. POSTMASTER: Send address changes to *Surgical Clinics*, Elsevier Health Sciences Division, Subscription Customer Service, 3251 Riverport Lane, Maryland Heights, MO 63043. **Customer Service (orders, claims, online, change of address): Telephone: 1-800-654-2452 (U.S. and Canada); 314-447-8871 (outside U.S. and Canada). Fax: 314-447-8029. E-mail: journalscustomerservice-usa@elsevier.com (for print support); journalsonline support-usa@elsevier.com (for online support).**

Reprints. For copies of 100 or more, of articles in this publication, please contact the Commercial Reprints Department, Elsevier Inc., 360 Park Avenue South, New York, New York 10010-1710. Tel. (212) 633-3812, Fax: (212) 462-1935, e-mail: reprints@elsevier.com.

The Surgical Clinics of North America is also published in Spanish by McGraw-Hill Interamericana Editores S.A., P.O. Box 5-237 06500 Mexico D.F. Mexico; and in Portuguese by Interlivros Edicoes Ltda., Rua Comandante Coelho 1085, CEP 21250, Rio de Janeiro, Brazil; and in Greek by Paschalidis Medical Publications, Athens Greece.

The Surgical Clinics of North America is covered in *MEDLINE/PubMed (Index Medicus), EMBASE/Excerpta Medica, Current Contents/Clinical Medicine, Current Contents/Life Sciences, Science Citation Index*, and *ISI/BIOMED*.

Printed and bound by CPI Group (UK) Ltd, Croydon, CR0 4YY

Transferred to Digital Print 2011

Contributors

CONSULTING EDITOR

RONALD F. MARTIN, MD
Staff Surgeon, Department of Surgery, Marshfield Clinic, Marshfield, Wisconsin; Clinical Associate Professor, University of Wisconsin School of Medicine and Public Health, Madison, Wisconsin; Colonel, Medical Corps, United States Army Reserve

GUEST EDITOR

GEORGE M. FUHRMAN, MD
Program Director, Department of Surgery, Atlanta Medical Center, Atlanta, Georgia

AUTHORS

WILLIAM C. BECK, MD
General Surgery Resident, Division of General Surgery, Department of Surgery, Vanderbilt University Medical Center, Vanderbilt University, Nashville, Tennessee

JOHN S. BOLTON, MD
Chairman, Department of Surgery Ochsner Clinic Foundation, New Orleans, Louisiana; Professor of Surgery, The University of Queensland School of Medicine–Ochsner Clinical School, Brisbane, Australia

ALFREDO M. CARBONELL II, DO, FACS, FACOS
Associate Professor of Clinical Surgery, Chief, Division of Minimal Access and Bariatric Surgery, Greenville Hospital System University Medical Center, University of South Carolina School of Medicine, Greenville, South Carolina

AARON CARR, MD
General Surgery Resident, General Surgery Residency Program, Atlanta Medical Center, Graduate Medical Education, Atlanta, Georgia

W. CHARLES CONWAY II, MD
Department of Surgery Ochsner Clinic Foundation, New Orleans, Louisiana

STEPHEN A. DADA, MD
Chief Resident, Department of Surgery, Atlanta Medical Center, Atlanta, Georgia

NATALIE DONN, BS
The Center for Surgical Digestive Disorders, Tampa General Hospital; Division of General Surgery, College of Medicine, University of South Florida, Tampa, Florida

GEORGE M. FUHRMAN, MD
Program Director, Department of Surgery, Atlanta Medical Center, Atlanta, Georgia

VALERIE P. GRIGNOL, MD
Resident in General Surgery, Department of Surgery, Wright State University Boonshoft School of Medicine, Miami Valley Hospital, Dayton, Ohio

DAVID A. KOOBY, MD
Associate Professor of Surgery, Division of Surgical Oncology, Department of Surgery, Winship Cancer Institute, Emory University, Atlanta, Georgia

CONSTANCE W. LEE, MD
General Surgery Resident, Department of Surgery, University of Florida College of Medicine, Gainesville, Florida

KENNETH LUBERICE, BS
The Center for Surgical Digestive Disorders, Tampa General Hospital; Division of General Surgery, College of Medicine, University of South Florida, Tampa, Florida

TAM T. MAI, MD
General Surgery Resident, Department of Surgery, University of South Alabama College of Medicine, Mobile, Alabama

SAMEER H. PATEL, MD
Research Fellow, Division of Surgical Oncology, Department of Surgery, Winship Cancer Institute, Emory University, Atlanta, Georgia

HAROLD PAUL, BS
The Center for Surgical Digestive Disorders, Tampa General Hospital; Division of General Surgery, College of Medicine, University of South Florida, Tampa, Florida

PHILIP T. RAMSAY, MD
General and Trauma Surgery, Surgical Critical Care, General Surgery Residency Program Faculty, General Surgery Residency Program, Atlanta Medical Center, Graduate Medical Education, Atlanta, Georgia

WILLIAM O. RICHARDS, MD, FACS
Professor and Chairman, Department of Surgery, University of South Alabama College of Medicine, Mobile, Alabama

ALEXANDER S. ROSEMURGY, MD
The Center for Surgical Digestive Disorders, Tampa General Hospital, Tampa, Florida

SHARONA B. ROSS, MD
The Center for Surgical Digestive Disorders, Tampa General Hospital; Division of General Surgery, College of Medicine, University of South Florida, Tampa, Florida

JACK W. ROSTAS III, MD
General Surgery Resident, Department of Surgery, University of South Alabama College of Medicine, Mobile, Alabama

GEORGE A. SAROSI Jr, MD
Associate Professor of Surgery, Robert H. Hux MD Professor of Surgery, Surgery Residency Program Director, Vice Chairman for Education, Department of Surgery, University of Florida College of Medicine; Assistant Chief of Surgical Service, NF/SG Veterans Affairs Medical Center, Gainesville, Florida

KENNETH W. SHARP, MD
Professor of Surgery, Chief, Division of General Surgery, Department of Surgery, Vanderbilt University Medical Center, Vanderbilt University, Nashville, Tennessee

PAULA M. TERMUHLEN, MD
Associate Professor of Surgery, Chief, Division of Surgical Oncology, Department of Surgery, Wright State University Boonshoft School of Medicine, Miami Valley Hospital, Dayton, Ohio

Contents

Foreword: Gastric Surgery **ix**

Ronald F. Martin

Preface: Gastric Surgery **xiii**

George M. Fuhrman

Gastric Acid and Digestive Physiology **977**

Philip T. Ramsay and Aaron Carr

The primary function of the stomach is to prepare food for digestion and absorption by the intestine. Acid production is the unique and central component of the stomach's contribution to the digestive process. Acid bathes the food bolus while stored in the stomach, facilitating digestion. An intact defense against mucosal damage by the stomach's acid is essential to avoid ulceration. This article focuses on the physiology of gastric acid production, the stomach's defense mechanisms against acid injury, and the most common challenges to the gastric defenses. A brief description of the stomach's nonacid digestive capabilities is included.

Gastric Motility Physiology and Surgical Intervention **983**

Jack W. Rostas III, Tam T. Mai, and William O. Richards

Disordered gastric motility represents a spectrum of dysfunction ranging from delayed gastric emptying to abnormally rapid gastric transit, commonly referred to as the "dumping syndrome." Both extremes of gastric motility disorders can arise from similar pathologic processes, and produce remarkably identical symptoms. This fact underscores the need to attain a precise diagnosis to ensure the institution of optimal therapy. Disordered gastric motility is primarily managed with dietary modification followed by pharmacotherapy, as traditional surgical interventions tend to be fraught with complications. However, continued improvements in minimally invasive diagnostic and therapeutic modalities promise novel options for earlier and more effective treatment.

Emergency Ulcer Surgery **1001**

Constance W. Lee and George A. Sarosi Jr

The rate of elective surgery for peptic ulcer disease has been declining steadily over the past 3 decades. During this same period, the rate of emergency ulcer surgery rose by 44%. This means that the gastrointestinal surgeon is likely to be called on to manage the emergent complications of peptic ulcer disease without substantial experience in elective peptic ulcer disease surgery. The goal of this review is to familiarize surgeons with our evolving understanding of the pathogenesis, epidemiology, presentation,

in 2010. As understanding of these tumors advances, rapid changes in recommendations will continue and should warrant regular updates in tumor management.

Minimally Invasive Gastric Surgery **1089**

Alfredo M. Carbonell II

The most common indications for gastric resection remain benign ulcer disease and neoplasm. Surgery for these diseases can be performed safely with laparoscopy. As surgeons adhere to the original tenets of open gastric resections while performing laparoscopic resections, disease outcomes will remain the same with the improved surgical outcomes of less pain, a shorter hospital stay, and a lower incidence of wound complications. Laparoscopic gastric resections can be divided into the more straightforward wedge/tumor resections performed for submucosal tumors or the more formal anatomic gastric resections. This article reviews the tools and techniques for laparoscopic gastric resection.

Postgastrectomy Syndromes **1105**

John S. Bolton and W. Charles Conway II

The first postgastrectomy syndrome was noted not long after the first gastrectomy was performed. The indications for gastric resection have changed dramatically over the past 4 decades, and the overall incidence of gastric resection has decreased. This article focuses on the small proportion of patients with severe, debilitating symptoms; these symptoms can challenge the acumen of the surgeon who is providing the patient's long-term follow-up and care. The article does not deal with the sequelae of bariatric surgery.

Miscellaneous Disorders and Their Management in Gastric Surgery: Volvulus, Carcinoid, Lymphoma, Gastric Varices, and Gastric Outlet Obstruction **1123**

Stephen A. Dada and George M. Fuhrman

This article focuses on less common diseases that surgeons are called on for management options. Five topics—volvulus, carcinoid, lymphoma, gastric varices, and gastric outlet obstruction from peptic ulcer disease—are frequently used to evaluate surgical knowledge. Knowledge of these topics is useful for residents preparing for an in-training examination or board certification. Patients with these diseases require multidisciplinary management with oncologists and/or gastroenterologists, and mastery of these topics allows surgeons to effectively participate in the multidisciplinary care of these patients and advocate for surgical management when appropriate.

Index **1131**

FORTHCOMING ISSUES

December 2011
Bariatric and Metabolic Surgery
Shanu Kothari, MD, *Guest Editor*

February 2012
Safe Surgery
Juan A. Sanchez, MD, MPA, FACS,
Guest Editor

April 2012
Management of Peri-operative Complications
Lewis J. Kaplan, MD, and
Stanley H. Rosenbaum, MD,
Guest Editors

June 2012
Pediatric Surgery
Kenneth S. Azarow, MD, and
Robert A. Cusick, MD,
Guest Editors

RECENT ISSUES

August 2011
Nutrition and Metabolism of The Surgical Patient, Part II
Stanley J. Dudrick, MD, and
Juan A. Sanchez, MD,
Guest Editors

June 2011
Nutrition and Metabolism of The Surgical Patient, Part I
Stanley J. Dudrick, MD, and
Juan A. Sanchez, MD, *Guest Editors*

April 2011
Update on Surgical Palliative Care
Geoffrey P. Dunn, MD, FACS,
Guest Editor

February 2011
Diagnostic Imaging for the General Surgeon
Thomas H. Cogbill, MD, and
Benjamin T. Jarman, MD,
Guest Editors

ISSUE OF RELATED INTEREST

Gastroenterology Clinics of North America September 2010 (Vol. 39, Issue 3)
Clinical Pharmacology of Gastrointestinal and Liver Disease
Richard H. Hunt, FRCP, FRCPEd, FRCPC, FACG, AGAF, *Guest Editor*

THE CLINICS ARE NOW AVAILABLE ONLINE!

Access your subscription at:
www.theclinics.com

Foreword
Gastric Surgery

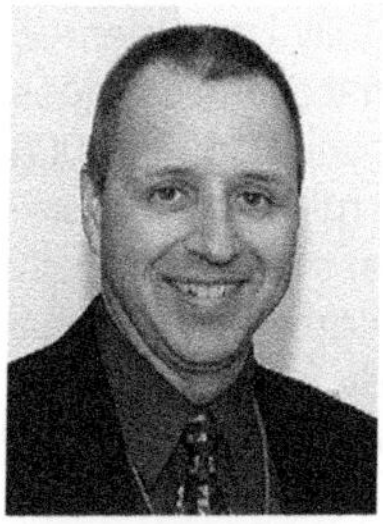

Ronald F. Martin, MD
Consulting Editor

Generally speaking, the forewords to each issue of the *Surgical Clinics of North America* are written with the intent of informing the reader as to why we have incorporated this particular set of topics into the series. For most surgeons it would appear somewhat self-evident as to the importance of the topic of Gastric Surgery to the overall understanding one must have to be a competent general surgeon. With that in mind, I should not like to insult the reader's intelligence by restating the obvious, but rather use this opportunity to consider what other examples we may take from this theme that might help us on larger questions. Two particular topics come to mind: the evolution of inquiry, and facts trumping beliefs.

I have written before, and still maintain, that the evolution of understanding of gastric anatomy and physiology, coupled with our ability to alter both structure and function by operative and nonoperative means, may be the best example of how surgeons think when they think best. I harbor no desire to belittle any of the contributions of other surgical endeavors, such as cardiac surgery, operative orthopedics, neurosurgery, operative endoscopy, or any of the others, but still, in my opinion, the development of gastric surgery is our crown jewel. The reasons are many-fold perhaps, but among them are its development was more-or-less first and therefore set the stage for many to follow in terms of intellectual rigor. Also, the principles studied have been reevaluated and modified and tested by means that we could measure fairly accurately. Last, but not exhaustively, we have modified and corrected our approach based upon changing circumstances and new technology, both operative and pharmaceutical, from the very beginning of the study of these topics in the latter 1800s. We have let ourselves be guided by facts inasmuch as we could understand them.

So we now find ourselves in 2011. In particular, we find ourselves in 2011 in the month of July at the writing of this foreword. What is peculiar about this month may not be evident to all, but the discipline of surgery in the United States has just experienced perhaps the most seismic event it has seen for some time. We have created two fundamentally distinct classes of surgical residents: those who can only work shifts of

Surg Clin N Am 91 (2011) ix–xi
doi:10.1016/j.suc.2011.07.002

0039-6109/11/$ – see front matter © 2011 Elsevier Inc. All rights reserved.

significantly less than one day and those who can follow patients clinically overnight. We now have PGY-1 residents who can no longer work more than 16 hours consecutively.

Some may argue that we created a "shift-work" model in 2003 in response to the initial Institute of Medicine report "To Err is Human." To be fair, some changes were proposed then but, if we are honest, many programs have still not fully implemented them and others have blurred many lines. One inescapable tidbit is that all the changes that were made in the stated guidelines for residency education conditions in 2003 were aimed at all resident levels and not just one subset. These new rules to be implemented this month create a class of learner (in our current parlance) that is not really a medical student and not really a resident. Perhaps we have lengthened medical school? Hard to argue that successfully since degrees have already been conferred prior to the learner arriving at the residency program and, furthermore, residency programs are completely regulated by the ACGME (Accreditation Council for Graduate Medical Education). The other characterization is that we have shortened residency. Many will argue that we haven't done that because it still takes five years (minimum) to complete a general surgery residency. Personally, that argument seems specious to me as we absolutely lose time in training PGY 1 residents under conditions that would qualify one as a resident in all the other resident years that we never get back. That leaves the ultimate conclusion that more time and transition to increased responsibility has to be compressed into the last 4 years of general surgical residency. And since time is what time is—just ask Einstein—time cannot be compressed here on Earth and residency training is at least functionally shorter.

So we have changed residency, at least in its first year, such that mandating time away from clinical experience is considered to be preferable to allowing continued observation for training superior surgeons. That is an interesting proposition. We should test it. But we won't.

If the above were true, we would expect a decrease in measurable complications. We might also expect an increase in some standardized test scores such as the American Board of Surgery (ABS) Qualifying Exam (QE) or the ABS Certifying Exam (CE). Perhaps we would get feedback from partners of newly graduated Chief Residents and Fellows that our newest additions to the nonsupervised work force were better prepared.

While we cannot yet assess the new PGY-1 rules, we can look at the interval since the 2003 rules changed, to whatever degree they were implemented. One can look at the published results of the ABS and see that the pass rates for first-time CE candidates is falling somewhat dramatically. The QE first-time pass rates may be harder to interpret based on the nature of assigning a passing grade is already subjected to a curve. Feedback to the Fellowship of the American College of Surgeons through its Board of Governors has suggested that there is increasing concern among hirers of recent graduates that our newly "independent" surgeons are not as prepared to practice independently as their predecessors. And, at least in my institution, where I supervise a Morbidity and Mortality conference, we are seeing an increase in and a greater proportion of what we believe to be preventable errors as a result of handing off responsibility and ownership of a patient's care between individuals. One caveat on this last bit is that it appears to be more attributable to handoffs between staff and faculty surgeons than resident surgeons. Still, it appears to us that failure of continuity is more dangerous than fatigue, although I cannot prove that at this time. I have not found good evidence that states we are producing better surgeons or getting better outcomes because of the changes, although it may be out there beyond my reach.

Many claims have been made along the way about the need for these changes; some of them wise and some of them not so wise. The least wise claim is the one that alleges that it is *impossible* to train competent surgeons under the "old" system. Unfortunately for proponents of that argument, we have nearly a century of surgical training and innovation that refutes that claim. Whether one likes or doesn't like the method by which those people were trained, it is irrefutable that they were trained and much of what we know was discovered by them. Perhaps the wisest claim is, the old system, or its recent iterations, is not desirable, as it does not *produce our best surgeons*. That is an interesting hypothesis that we should be able to test.

So back to gastric surgery: what Dr Fuhrman and his colleagues have done is given the reader a fresh look at a long-studied and thought to be well-understood area of surgery and medicine. Fresh looks are good. So good that we at *Surgical Clinics* always get a different guest editor when we revisit a topic. Through this fresh look we get a chance to see if our long-held assumptions still withstand scrutiny and if the current facts still support our beliefs.

We surgeons should be encouraged by our history and should demand of our professional organizations, such as the American College of Surgeons, the American Board of Surgery, the Review Committee for Surgery, and the multitude of societies and other boards, that the proposed changes in training our future partners, and, perhaps as importantly, our own future surgeons (remember—everybody is preop, including us), should be designed and implemented with the expressed intent of testing these changes to see if they produce the desired goal. And if they don't, we should modify the situation accordingly.

There should be plans to assess whether these changes make the world a safer place for the patient or community by measurements that we can agree upon. There should be nodes in the decision plot that allow us to modify our trajectory of change, or even go back, if we find that our changes have made matters worse. And perhaps most importantly, we must be able to assess if a "best practice" model to train one specialty group of physicians is also the best for other specialties. We may find that a model that works best for pathologists is different than that for primary care or anesthesiologists or surgeons. In fact, I would be shocked if we didn't.

At present, these changes are made by fiat on questionable grounds largely about the impact of training schedules on the individual trainee and not about the impact of the future trainee on society. And at the end of the day, it is not about us—it is about the patient. We surgeons have historically prided ourselves on being leaders for the causes of our patients. Should we not do that now?

Ronald F. Martin, MD
Department of Surgery
Marshfield Clinic
1000 North Oak Avenue
Marshfield, WI 54449, USA

E-mail address:
Martin.ronald@marshfieldclinic.org

Preface
Gastric Surgery

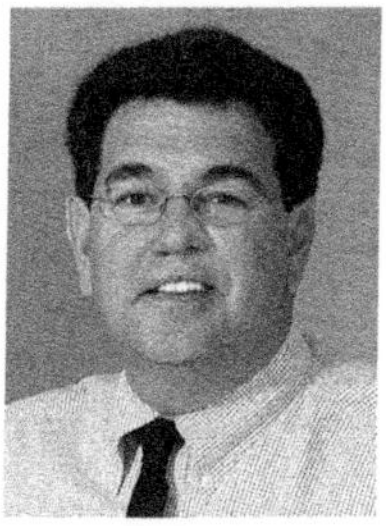

George M. Fuhrman, MD
Guest Editor

I appreciate the opportunity to serve as guest editor for this issue of *Surgical Clinics of North America*. As the second decade of my surgical career nears its end, I have had the opportunity to manage many patients with all of the diseases included in this issue and take great pleasure in trying to restore their ability to eat and improve their quality of life by achieving independence from central hyperalimentation and feeding tubes. I have tried to balance this issue with both basic science and clinical information necessary for developing a sophisticated appreciation for gastric pathophysiology.

The authors included in this issue represent three important groups of surgeons. First, I have asked several senior surgeons that have contributed to my training through their direct teaching, writings, and presentations at national meetings. They are each masters in the field of gastrointestinal surgery and add an element of sophistication to this edition. The authors also include a group of mid-career surgeons for whom I have great admiration. The quality of their articles is extraordinary. They are the future giants in the field of gastrointestinal surgery. Finally, several members of my current department of surgery, both faculty and trainees, have participated in the creation of this issue. While their names are likely to be unfamiliar to the reader, each has provided me with great surgical insight through their questions in conferences, on rounds, and in the operating room. They come to work each day with a high level of intellectual curiosity that stimulates my desire to learn and teach.

George M. Fuhrman, MD
Department of Surgery
Atlanta Medical Center, Box 423
303 Parkway, NE
Atlanta, GA 30312, USA

E-mail address:
george.fuhrman@tenethealth.com

Surg Clin N Am 91 (2011) xiii
doi:10.1016/j.suc.2011.06.013
0039-6109/11/$ – see front matter © 2011 Elsevier Inc. All rights reserved.

Gastric Acid and Digestive Physiology

Philip T. Ramsay, MD*, Aaron Carr, MD

KEYWORDS

• Gastric acid • Stomach • Digestive physiology

The primary function of the stomach is to prepare food for digestion and absorption by the intestine. Although various neural and hormonal mediators contribute to gastric function, acid production is the unique and central component of the stomach's contribution to the digestive process. Liquids pass easily through the stomach and into the small intestine. Solid components remain in the stomach until they are small enough to be slowly released into the small intestine by the coordinated action of the antrum and pylorus. Acid bathes the food bolus while stored in the stomach, facilitating digestion. An intact defense against mucosal damage by the stomach's acid is essential to avoid ulceration. This article focuses on the physiology of gastric acid production, the stomach's defense mechanisms against acid injury, and the most common challenges to the gastric defenses. A brief description of the stomach's nonacid digestive capabilities is included.

THE PROTON PUMP

The mucosa of the gastric body, and to a lesser extent the fundus and antrum, contains the parietal cells. One function of the parietal cell is to produce gastric acid, which activates pepsin from pepsinogen, aids in the digestion of protein, and reduces bacterial colonization of the stomach and duodenum.[1] The parietal cell contains the hydrogen (H^+)/potassium (K^+)-ATPase, or proton pump, which transports H^+ out of the cell into the gastric lumen and K^+ from the gastric lumen into the cell.[2] Interestingly, the H+ gradient created in the gastric lumen is greater than 10^6 times that of blood.[3] Because of the large amount of energy needed to run the proton pump, the parietal cell has the largest mitochondrial capacity of any cell in the human body.[1] In the resting parietal cell, the proton pumps are contained within the membranes of intracellular tubulovesicles.[3] There is a constant basal level of acid production, even in the unstimulated parietal cell.[1] The basal level of acid secretion is caused by histamine and acetylcholine.[4] Basal acid output is approximately 10% of the maximal acid output of the stimulated parietal cell. There is diurnal

General Surgery Residency Program, Atlanta Medical Center, Graduate Medical Education, 303 Parkway Drive, North East, Atlanta, GA 30312, USA
* Corresponding author.
E-mail address: ptrams@hotmail.com

Surg Clin N Am 91 (2011) 977–982
doi:10.1016/j.suc.2011.06.010 surgical.theclinics.com
0039-6109/11/$ – see front matter © 2011 Elsevier Inc. All rights reserved.

variation of basal acid levels, with night levels being higher than day levels.[1] In the stimulated state, the tubulovesicles fuse with the apical cell membrane, thus relocating the proton pumps to the apical surface of the parietal cell.[1,3] The apical cell membrane also contains cotransport channels for K^+ and chloride (Cl^-), which transport both K^+ and Cl^- out of the cell into the gastric lumen. Therefore, there is a net transfer of H^+ and Cl^- into the gastric lumen with stimulation of the proton pump.[2]

PARIETAL CELL RECEPTORS

There are three stimulatory receptors on the parietal cell: the muscarinic (M_3) receptor, the type B cholecystokinin (CCK_B) receptor, and the histamine (H_2) receptor (**Fig. 1**).[3] These receptors are located on the basolateral membranes of the parietal cell.[4] The M_3 receptor is stimulated by acetylcholine and activates gastric acid secretion by an intracellular calcium (Ca^{2+}) pathway that increases intracellular Ca^{2+} levels.[3] Acetylcholine is released from the stimulation of parasympathetic vagal nerve fibers.[1]

The CCK_B receptor, or gastrin receptor, is stimulated by gastrin and also activates acid secretion by an intracellular Ca^{2+} pathway that increases intracellular Ca^{2+} levels.[3] The gastric antral mucosa, and to a lesser extent the duodenal mucosa, contains G cells, which produce gastrin.[1,4] Protein is the major stimulant for gastrin release.[1] Gastrin is produced in the endoplasmic reticulum and is released through the basal membrane of the G cell.[4] Vagal stimulation also causes the release of gastrin-releasing peptide (GRP), the equivalent to bombesin, from cells in the gastric fundal mucosa.[1,2,5] GRP then stimulates gastrin release from gastric antral G cells.[2] In addition to the stimulation of acid secretion, gastrin also has a trophic effect on both parietal cells and enterochromaffin-like (ECL) cells.[1]

The H_2 receptor is stimulated by histamine and activates acid secretion by a pathway that increases intracellular cAMP.[3] Histamine is produced by ECL cells, and its release is stimulated by gastrin and acetylcholine.[1] The stimulatory effect of acetylcholine and gastrin is thought to occur through or in combination with histamine.[3] The final outcome from stimulation of the M_3, CCK_B, and H_2 receptors is the activation of the H^+/K^+-ATPase.[2] Activation of these receptors in any combination results in a greater amount of gastric acid release than with activation of any one of the receptors alone. This effect is known as potentiation[4]. To completely block

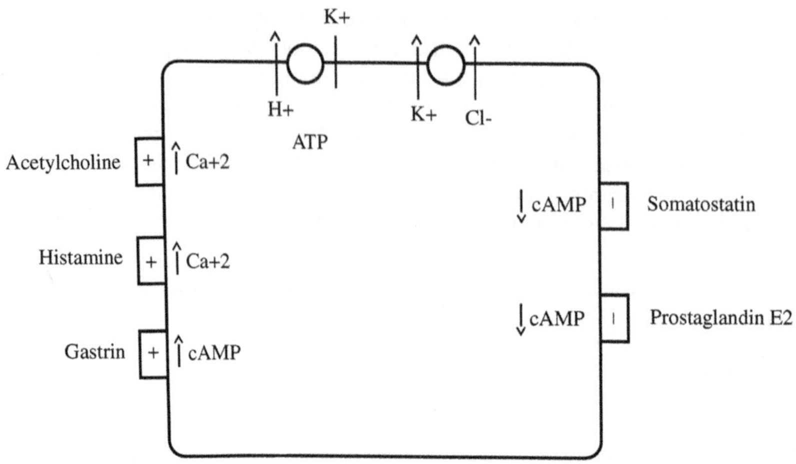

Fig. 1. The parietal cell.

stimulation of acid secretion through the activation of these receptors, all 3 receptors must be blocked individually.[2] However, the use of a proton pump inhibitor alone will block acid secretion by inhibiting the final common pathway, the H^+/K^+-ATPase itself.[1,2]

Somatostain is produced by D cells present in the fundic and antral mucosa and in the small intestine.[1,4] Somatostatin has an inhibitory effect on gastric acid release. Intraluminal acid has a stimulatory effect, and acetylcholine has an inhibitory effect on somatostatin release. Somatostatin not only inhibits the parietal cell directly, but also indirectly by inhibiting the release of gastrin and histamine.[1] Direct parietal cell inhibition occurs via the reduction of intracellular cAMP.[3]

The parietal cell also contains another inhibitory receptor for prostaglandin E_2 (PGE_2).[2] PGE_2 also inhibits gastric acid secretion by decreasing intracellular cAMP levels.[3,4] Additionally, PGE_2 inhibits gastrin secretion and stimulates somatostatin secretion.[4]

THE CEPHALIC, GASTRIC, AND INTESTINAL PHASES OF GASTRIC ACID SECRETION

Gastric acid secretion can be divided into 3 phases: the cephalic, gastric, and intestinal phases.[2] The cephalic phase of gastric acid secretion is mediated by vagal excitation stimulated by the thought, sight, smell, or taste of food.[1,2] This can be elicited by sham feeding. Vagal excitation causes the release of acetylcholine, which stimulates gastric acid and pepsin secretion from mucosal parietal cells and chief cells, respectively.[2]

The gastric phase of gastric acid secretion is mediated by gastric distention as food enters the gastric lumen.[1,2] The majority of gastric acid release occurs during this phase.[1] Gastric antral distention causes the release of gastrin from G cells. Distention of the gastric fundus increases the effects of gastrin and histamine through a local cholinergic pathway. Intraluminal acid inhibits the release of gastrin from G cells.[2]

The intestinal phase of gastric acid secretion is primarily inhibitory and begins when food enters the small intestine.[1,2] The least amount of gastric acid is released during this phase.[1] Intraintestinal acid inhibits gastric acid secretion through an enterogastrone.[2]

GASTRIC MUCUS, MUCOSAL DEFENSE, AND REPAIR

Mucus forms a protective layer over the gastric and duodenal mucosa.[2] Mucus is released by exocytosis from mucus neck cells and surface mucus cells in the stomach and Brunner glands in the duodenum.[2,5] Mucus contains mostly water and smaller amounts of electrolytes and mucin glycoproteins. Mucin glycoproteins make mucus a viscous gel. The main physiologic stimulus for the release of mucus is acetylcholine. Secretin also stimulates mucus secretion, and prostaglandins increase mucus viscosity and mucin glycoprotein content. Mucus slows the diffusion of acid from the gastric lumen to the gastric mucosa. Mucus also contains bicarbonate (HCO_3^-), which maintains a near-normal pH at the mucosal surface.[2] This is known as the unstirred layer.[1] HCO_3^- is secreted by both active and passive processes. Mucus also provides lubrication for the passage of food, thus protecting the mucosa from mechanical stresses. Mucus is not broken down by gastric acid, but it is dissolved by pepsin and N-acetylcysteine. It is easily penetrated by bile salts, ethanol, and nonsteroidal anti-inflammatory drugs (NSAIDs), which lead to mucosal injury.[2] Mucosal damage is caused by offensive agents or decreased defense.[1] After injury, a mucus layer is formed containing fibrin and dead cells over the site of injury. Degraded mucus is replaced by continuous mucus secretion.[2]

The apical membrane of the mucosal cell is impermeable to H^+. However, H^+ can diffuse between cell junctions to reach the basolateral surfaces of the cell. High concentrations of H^+ cause mucosal injury. The mucosa is protected from this by HCO_3^-. The basolateral surfaces of mucosal parietal cells regulate pH through an HCO_3^-/Cl^- antiporter. For every H^+ transported out of the cell through the apical membrane during acid secretion, an HCO_3^- is transported out of the cell through the basolateral membrane.[2] This phenomenon is known as the alkaline tide.[5] This neutralizes any H^+ that reaches the basolateral membranes. The HCO_3^-/Cl^- antiporter can also be activated by prostaglandins, even without the stimulation of acid secretion. The parietal cell basolateral membranes also contain an Na^+/H^+ antiporter that transports Na^+ into the cell and H^+ out of the cell. This transporter protects against intracellular acidosis. The driving force for this transporter is a basolateral Na^+/K^+-ATPase.[2]

After mucosal injury, rapid repair, or restitution, occurs within minutes.[1,2,5] Repair occurs through the movement of already established mature mucosal cells over the basal lamina.[2] Therefore, repair does not require the generation of new mucosal cells through cell division.[1,2] This is an important mechanism for repair of the mucosa after normal physiologic stresses. Repair can be impeded by luminal acid, calcium depletion, low HCO_3^-, and altered cell motility. Delayed repair results in the formation of ulcers.[2]

GASTRIC CIRCULATION

Vagal stimulation, through the action of acetylcholine, causes vasodilation of the gastric vasculature and increased blood flow. Histamine also causes vasodilation. Therefore, stimulation of acid secretion is associated with increases in gastric blood flow.[2] Endogenous nitric oxide (NO) and PGE_2 also cause vasodilation.[4] Sympathetic stimulation, as well as exogenous epinephrine, norepinephrine, and vasopressin, causes vasoconstriction of the gastric vasculature and decreased blood flow. Hemorrhagic shock leads to decreased blood flow and increased susceptibility of the gastric mucosa to injury by acid and bile salts. Aging is also associated with decreased blood flow. Agents that increase gastric blood flow have a protective effect on the stomach. The relationship between gastric blood flow and mucosal injury is due to the acid–base balance of the tissue. Adequate blood flow prevents tissue acidosis and mucosal injury. Autoregulatory mechanisms maintain a constant gastric blood flow with changes in arterial pressure up to a certain point.[2] Blood flow is an important component in gastric mucosal defense by delivering nutrients and oxygen to mucosal cells. Blood flow of 50% to 75% of normal leads to mucosal injury.[1]

PEPSIN

The chief cells synthesize and release the proenzyme pepsinogen, the precursor to pepsin[2]. The chief cells are the most abundant cells in the gastric mucosa. They are found in the body, fundus, and antrum of the stomach, as well as in the duodenum.[1] Pepsinogen is produced in the endoplasmic reticulum, and its release by exocytosis is stimulated by acetylcholine, histamine, and CCK.[2,4] Pepsinogen release is inhibited by somatostatin.[4] Active pepsin is formed in an acidic environment by cleavage of the N-terminal amino acid sequence of pepsinogen.[2] Pepsin, along with gastric acid, facilitates the digestion of protein.[5]

INTRINSIC FACTOR

An additional function of the parietal cell is the synthesis and secretion of intrinsic factor (IF).[2] IF is the only essential substance produced by the stomach.[5] It is necessary for adequate absorption of vitamin B_{12} (cyanocobalamin) in the terminal ileum.[1,2] IF is produced in the endoplasmic reticulum and is released from the apical surface of the parietal cell.[4] The same factors that stimulate the secretion of acid also stimulate the secretion of IF; however, acid secretion and IF secretion may not be linked.[2,5] The production of IF greatly exceeds that which is necessary for adequate absorption of cobalamin. Most patients manufacture adequate IF after subtotal gastrectomy, making vitamin B_{12} supplementation unnecessary.[2]

NSAIDs

NSAIDs cause damage to gastric mucosa by direct injury and by affecting prostaglandin production, specifically PGE_2.[2,6] NSAIDS are lipophilic weak acids; therefore they bind to gastric mucosa and induce local injury. Their major mechanism of action is systemic inhibition of cyclooxygenase (COX), an enzyme in the pathway of the production of prostaglandins from arachadonic acid. Two isoforms exist: COX 1 and COX 2. Nonselective NSAIDs block both isoforms, but selective inhibitors block only COX 2. The COX 1 pathway results in production of PGE_2. PGE_2 protects the gastric mucosa by decreasing gastric acid secretion, increasing mucus production and bicarbonate secretion, and increasing mucosal blood $flow_2$. The net effect of nonselective NSAIDS is reduction of prostaglandins (including PGE_2), which leads to mucosal injury. COX 2 is primarily expressed during inflammatory events, and the prostaglandins produced by this pathway promote the inflammatory response. Selective NSAIDS block COX 2 but have little effect on COX 1, which results in an anti-inflammatory effect without the deleterious effects on gastric mucosa. Synthetic PGE_2, or misoprostol, acts by inhibiting gastric acid secretion and enhanced mucosal protection.[6] This can be used in patients requiring long-term nonselective NSAIDS to prevent injury to gastrointestinal mucosa.[6,7] H2 blockers and proton pump inhibitors can also be used to reduce the risk of complications from nonselective NSAIDS.[7]

HELICOBACTER PYLORI

Helicobacter pylori is a gram-negative flagellated rod that possesses the enzyme urease. Urease converts urea into ammonia (NH_3) and carbon dioxide (CO_2), allowing the organism to survive in the low pH of the stomach. Colonization leads to gastric mucosal inflammation and injury.[8] *H pylori* also produces enzymes that break down mucus. In addition, patients with *H pylori* infection have a lower D cell population than those without infection. This leads to lower somatostatin levels, higher gastrin levels, and increased acid secretion. Only gastric mucosa, or gastric-type mucosa, contains receptors specific for *H pylori*.[1] Up to 50% of the population is infected with *H pylori*.[8] Patients infected with this organism may be asymptomatic or may develop antral gastritis, gastric or duodenal ulcers, or mucosa-associated lymphoid tissue (MALT) lymphoma.[1,2] Almost all cases of chronic antral gastritis and duodenal ulcers and most gastric ulcers are associated with *H pylori* infection.[9] Eradication of *H pylori* restores the D cell population with the resultant decrease in gastric acid secretion.[1] Treatment shortens the healing time of ulcers and decreases the chance of relapse.[2]

SUMMARY

Gastric acid physiology is a complex process involving the parasympathetic vagus nerve and a variety of hormones including gastrin, histamine, somatostatin, and prostaglandin. In addition to gastric acid, the stomach produces pepsin and intrinsic factor. The gastric mucosa is protected by mucus and bicarbonate secretion. Mucosal defense is adversely affected by *H pylori* infection and NSAIDs. Gastric acid production facilitates digestion; however, damage from excess acid or inadequate mucosal defense can result in ulceration.

REFERENCES

1. Mercer DW, Robinson EK. Stomach. In: Townsend CM, editor. Sabiston textbook of surgery. 18th edition. Philadelphia: Saunders; 2008. p. 1226–38.
2. Silen W. Physiology of gastric function. In: Fischer JE, editor. Surgical basic science. St Louis (MO): Mosby; 1993. p. 271–91.
3. Urushidani T, Forte JG. Signal transduction and activation of acid secretion in the parietal cell. J Membr Biol 1997;159:99–111.
4. Mulholland MW. Gastric anatomy and physiology. In: Mulholland MW, editor. Greenfield's surgery: scientific principles and practice. 4th edition. Philadelphia: Lippincott Williams and Wilkins; 2006. p. 712–20.
5. Dempsey DT. Stomach. In: Brunicardi FC, editor. Schwartz's principles of surgery. 9th edition. New York: McGraw-Hill; 2010. p. 894–9, 908.
6. Sostres S, Gargallo CJ, Arroyo MT, et al. Adverse effects of nonsteroidal anti-inflammatory drugs (NSAIDs, aspirin and Coxibs) on upper gastrointestinal tract. Best Pract Res Clin Gastroenterol 2010;24:121–32.
7. Rostom A, Muir K, Dube C, et al. Prevention of NSAID-related upper gastrointestinal toxicity: a meta-analysis of traditional NSAIDs with gastroprotection and COX-2 Inhibitors. Drug Healthc Patient Saf 2009;1:47–71.
8. Ryan KJ. Vibrio, campylobacter, and helicobacter. In: Ryan KJ, Ray CG, editors. Sherris medical microbiology. 4th edition. New York: McGraw-Hill; 2004. p. 381–2.
9. Liu C, Crawford JM. The gastrointestinal tract. In: Kumar V, Abbas AK, Fausto N, editors. Robbins and cotran pathologic basis of disease. 7th edition. Philadelphia: Elsevier; 2005. p. 813, 814, 817, 818.

Gastric Motility Physiology and Surgical Intervention

Jack W. Rostas III, MD, Tam T. Mai, MD, William O. Richards, MD*

KEYWORDS

- Gastric motility • Physiology • Delayed gastric emptying
- Gastroparesis • Dumping syndrome
- Gastric electrical stimulation

The stomach plays a critical role in digestion, as a site of significant processing of meals and distribution of chyme to the small intestine. Gastric motility requires extensive integration of neural and hormonal regulatory input, rendering proper function vulnerable to a host of pathologic processes. Disordered gastric function can manifest as a spectrum of symptoms, ranging from inconvenient to completely debilitating and potentially life threatening. Whereas symptomatic gastric dysmotility is managed nonoperatively in the majority of cases, surgical intervention is required for patients with severe symptoms refractory to medical therapy. Therefore, the foregut surgeon must be thoroughly familiar with the current diagnostic and management techniques available for deranged gastric motility.

NORMAL GASTRIC MOTILITY

Background

The traditional anatomic structures of the stomach are the fundus, corpus (body), antrum, and pylorus. These anatomically distinct regions do not correlate with the functional regions of the stomach.[1] In general, the proximal stomach serves as a temporary reservoir for meals, while the distal stomach churns and mixes food with digestive juices. Once the distal stomach has processed the solid food to an appropriate size and consistency, the pylorus regulates its outflow into the duodenum. The proximal reservoir consists of the fundus and proximal one-third of the corpus, the distal pump consists of the distal two-thirds of the corpus and antrum, and the pyloric sphincter comprises the final gate to the small bowel[2] (**Fig. 1**[3]).

Gastric smooth muscle activity is modulated by myogenic, neural, and hormonal influences. Intrinsic myogenic contraction forms the fundamental basis of gastric

The authors have nothing to disclose.
Department of Surgery, University of South Alabama College of Medicine, 2451 Fillingim Street, Mobile, AL 36617, USA
* Corresponding author.
E-mail address: brichards@usouthal.edu

Surg Clin N Am 91 (2011) 983–999
doi:10.1016/j.suc.2011.06.012
surgical.theclinics.com
0039-6109/11/$ – see front matter © 2011 Elsevier Inc. All rights reserved.

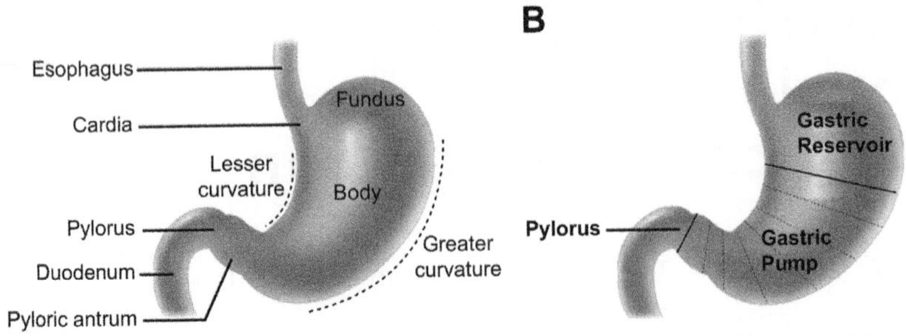

Fig. 1. Anatomic and functional regions of the stomach. (*A*) Anatomic regions. (*B*) Functional regions. (*Adapted from* Mercer DW, Liu TH, Castaneda A. Anatomy and physiology of the stomach. In: Zuidema GD, Yeo CJ. Shackelford's surgery of the alimentary tract. 5th edition, vol. 2. Philadelphia: Saunders; 2002. p. 3. Copyright Elsevier; with permission.)

motility, and occurs in the absence of any other influence.[2] Neural regulation emanates primarily from the intrinsic gastric myenteric plexus, with further contributions from extrinsic parasympathetic (vagal) and sympathetic (splanchnic) input.[4] Hormonal influences play a significant role in the regulation of gastric motility. The list of hormones known to modulate gastric motility is extensive (**Table 1**[5–10]).

Gastric peristalsis occurs primarily in the distal stomach and is regulated by the gastric slow wave, a 3-cycle-per-minute depolarization of the smooth muscle cell membrane.[4] The gastric slow waves are paced by the interstitial cells of Cajal (ICC), specialized cells located primarily along the mid-portion of the greater curvature of the stomach. The ICC provide the coordination and propagation of electrical activity within the gastric smooth muscle cells.[4] The propagation of the slow wave is slightly faster in the greater curvature as compared with the lesser curvature, such that the signals synchronize on reaching the pylorus.[11]

Fasting Gastric Motility

Fasting gastric motility comprises the migrating motor complex (MMC), which serves to clear indigested debris from the lumen of the stomach and intestine.[2] During this period the proximal stomach undergoes tonic contraction, while the gastric slow wave modulates the coordinated peristalsis of the distal stomach.[4] The MMC consists of a 90- to 120-minute cycle with 4 distinct phases. Phase I comprises a 40- to 60-minute period of inactivity. Phase II is heralded by the progressive but irregular increase in the magnitude of the peristaltic wave over a period of 30 to 50 minutes. Phase III consists of high-amplitude, regular contractions at 3 cycles per minute over a 5- to 10-minute period, which performs the task of clearing luminal contents. The pylorus is open for the duration of this phase to allow emptying. Phase IV marks the rapid return to baseline from the contractions during phase III (**Fig. 2**[12]).

Postprandial Gastric Motility

Five to 10 minutes after the ingestion of food the MMC gives way to the fed state of gastric muscle activity.[2,4] The proximal stomach stretches to accommodate the contents of a meal and allow mixing of gastric contents with pepsin and hydrochloric acid to initiate digestion. Relaxation of the proximal gastric smooth muscle occurs in response to swallowing, a reflex termed "receptive relaxation." Similarly, expansion of the proximal stomach occurs in response to increases in gastric volume, a process referred to as "gastric accommodation." These processes occur via stimulatory vagal input, as well as intrinsic and vasovagal reflexes in response to stretch. The overall

Table 1
Hormonal influences of gastric motility

	Stimulation	Site of Secretion	Other Actions
Stimulatory Hormone			
Gastrin	Gastric pH >3, vagus nerve, antral distention, protein, calcium, alcohol	Gastric antrum and duodenum (G cells)	Inhibits small bowel and colonic motility
Ghrelin	Fasting	Gastric fundus	Stimulates hunger
Motilin	Acid and vagus nerve	Stomach and duodenum (M cells)	Induces phase 3 MMC duodenal peristalsis
Inhibitory Hormone			
Cholecystokinin	Increased fat and protein in small bowel	Duodenum and jejunum	Gastric relaxation, sensation of fullness
Glucagon	Hypoglycemia, amino acids, β-adrenergic stimulation	Pancreas (α cells)	Slows MMC
Glucagon-like peptide 1	Increased glucose, fatty acids, and amino acids	Distal small intestine and colon	Decreases appetite
Peptide YY	Increased glucose, fatty acids, and amino acids	Terminal ileum and colon	Decreases appetite
Secretin	Acid, lipid, or bile in duodenal lumen	Duodenum (D cells)	Acts indirectly via inhibiting gastrin release
Somatostatin	Acidification of duodenal lumen	Gastric antrum (D cells)	Induces fasting small intestinal activity

Data from Refs.[5–10]

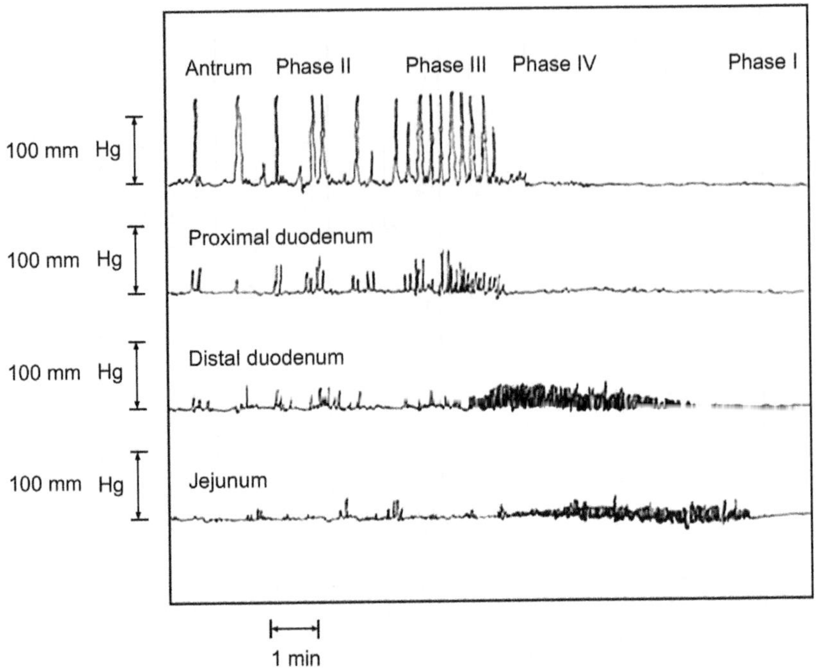

Fig. 2. Migrating motility complex of the distal stomach. Contraction of the gastric antrum increases in frequency approaching phase III, at which time clearing of the gastric lumen occurs before the return to the quiescent state of phase IV. The peristaltic activity of the gastric antrum is shown progressing to the duodenum and jejunum. (*From* Rees WD, Malagelada JR, Miller LJ, et al. Human interdigestive and postprandial gastrointestinal motor and gastrointestinal hormone patterns. Dig Dis Sci 1982;27:323. Copyright Springer Science+Business Media; with permission.)

result is expansion of the proximal stomach to provide temporary storage for the contents of a meal, without an increase in intragastric pressure.[2]

In the presence of food, the myenteric plexus releases hormonal signals to stimulate the gastric membrane potential to undergo an absolute increase in magnitude.[4] On reaching threshold potential, an action potential results and contraction occurs in the distal stomach. Neurotransmitters from extrinsic neurons modulate the amplitude of action potentials in a dose-dependent manner. Acetylcholine, released from the vagus nerve, functions as an excitatory neurotransmitter, while the inhibitory neurotransmitters norepinephrine, nitric oxide, and vasoactive intestinal peptide are withheld from release from splanchnic neurons.[1]

Peristalsis begins at the mid-stomach at the site of the gastric pacemaker and progresses along the body toward the pylorus, mobilizing and crushing food into a particulate consistency to facilitate its passage distally. Initially, contractions of irregular magnitude and frequency originate in the distal stomach. This pattern is similar to phase II of the MMC, with the exception that only about half of the gastric slow-wave potentials reach threshold for contraction. During each contraction, luminal contents lag behind the progression of the peristaltic wave, due to frictional forces against the gastric wall. Larger particles are forced retrograde to be exposed to these frictional forces repeatedly until adequately reduced in size. This effect is more pronounced with the more solid component of the chyme mixture.

The distal most portion of the stomach is the pylorus, a thick muscular ring that serves to regulate bidirectional passage of material between the antrum and duodenum. The peristaltic wave leads to a narrowing of the pylorus at the leading edge of the admixture, allowing only liquids and particulate matter 1 to 2 mm in size to funnel appropriately out of the stomach. The pylorus remains closed for most of the duration of the fed state, synchronized with the most intense antral contractions to facilitate churning of food. Opening occurs intermittently in conjunction with relatively minor antral contractions, to allow passage of processed gastric contents.

Gastric Emptying

Strict regulation of gastric motility ensures the appropriate delivery of gastric contents into the duodenum to allow for optimal absorption.[1] This process requires passage of gastric contents at both the appropriate rate and composition. The regulation of gastric emptying begins with the accommodation of the proximal stomach. This expansion in response to a food bolus allows timely flow to the distal stomach for processing and distribution. Abnormally reduced compliance of the proximal stomach results in increased intragastric pressure and accelerated emptying. Normal transit allows gastric contents to pass from the proximal to the distal stomach for processing and, in conjunction with the pylorus, delivery to the small bowel.

The composition of the gastric contents affects the rate of gastric emptying. Liquid emptying occurs more rapidly than that of solids, and is completed first when both are present. However, the emptying time of liquids increases with the relative proportion of the solid component. Solid emptying initially occurs slowly to allow for mixing and processing of gastric contents, and increases progressively as smaller particles become available for emptying. Solid-phase gastric emptying, as measured by the technetium-99–labeled scrambled egg study, classically demonstrates a 10- to 20-minute lag phase corresponding to the grinding of food, which is followed by a linear emptying of the food into the duodenum. Gastric emptying of liquids does not show the lag phase, as liquids exit the pylorus via first-order kinetics, directly proportional to the volume present[1] (**Fig. 3**[13]). This exit translates into a normal gastric emptying time of approximately 120 minutes, or a $T_{1/2}$ of 60 to 90 minutes, after an average, mixed solid/liquid meal.

The gastric emptying rate is primarily governed by caloric content, to allow for optimal absorption in the small intestine. The rate of gastric emptying is tightly regulated to distribute 1 to 4 kilocalories per minute to the proximal small bowel.[5] Consequently, fats empty slower than either carbohydrates or proteins. Cholecystokinin (CCK) plays a pivotal role in this process via inhibition of gastric emptying. CCK is released from the small intestine in the presence of intraluminal fat and protein.[1] Other characteristics of the gastric contents that determine emptying rate include anxiety, fear, depression, and intense exercise. Decreased temperature of the luminal contents also delays emptying, whereas the converse is true for increased temperature.[14,15] Hypertonic or hypotonic contents exit more slowly than isotonic solutions.

Similar to the stomach, the duodenum contains an intrinsically regulated pacing system. However, the duodenal slow wave frequency is regulated at 12 cycles per minute. Therefore, the gastric peristaltic wave approaches the gastroduodenal junction and synchronizes with only about one-fourth of the duodenal contractions.[11] This frequent, independent peristalsis ensures clearance of the duodenal lumen for efficient reception of gastric contents.

The gastrointestinal (GI) tract distal to the stomach also has multiple processes in place to regulate the flow of gastric contents. The duodenum and colon partially regulate their own inflow when distended, via a reflex arc that results in decreased fundal

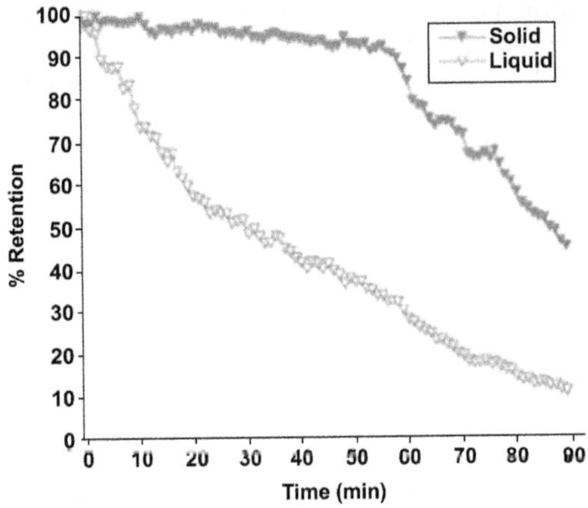

Fig. 3. Gastric emptying of solids and liquids. Gastric emptying of a solid meal (*filled triangles*) demonstrates a delay during the lag phase, followed by a linear emptying phase. Liquid emptying (*open triangles*) exhibits first-order kinetics without the initial lag phase. (*From* Hellström PM, Grybäck P, Jacobsson H. The physiology of gastric emptying. Best Pract Res Clin Anaesthesiol 2006;20(3):400; with permission.)

tone.[4] The duodenum also directly contracts to slow filling in response to stretch. The presence of high concentrations of glucose, lipids, or protein in the lumen of the ileum slows gastric emptying. This reflex, termed the "ileal brake," is largely induced by the release of peptide YY from the ileum.[16] A similar process occurs in the duodenum in response to lipid and protein. These components of GI regulation serve to further optimize the flow rate of nutrients into the distal bowel to maximize the absorptive capacity of the intestine.[2]

DISORDERS OF GASTRIC MOTILITY

The complex mechanisms influencing gastric motility allow a wide number of pathologic processes to interfere with normal transit. Disorders of gastric motility fall under the Rome III consensus criteria of functional dyspepsia, in the subcategory of postprandial distress syndrome.[17] These criteria represents a spectrum of dysfunction ranging from abnormally slow transit, termed delayed gastric emptying (DGE), to abnormally rapid gastric emptying, commonly referred to as "dumping syndrome." Although divergent in origin, both rapid and delayed gastric emptying can produce remarkably similar symptoms.[18] Varying degrees of nausea, vomiting, and abdominal pain can be the predominant symptoms in both extremes of gastric motility disorders, although the presence of diarrhea is more likely to occur in rapid emptying.[19] To further complicate matters, both of these divergent disorders can result from diabetes or vagal nerve dysfunction.[19] These similarities emphasize the importance of obtaining a precise history and physical examination during evaluation. Correctly distinguishing these two processes is critical in ensuring the proper application of what is often quite divergent therapy.

DGE is typified by diabetic gastroparesis, while rapid emptying is best exemplified by the classic postsurgical "dumping syndrome." The presence of any related symptoms merits a complete investigation, to establish the proper diagnosis and its underlying cause. Fortunately, these disorders overwhelmingly stem from benign processes, such as diabetes and postsurgical alterations. However, the etiology must be firmly established to ensure that a more concerning disease, such as a systemic autoimmune disorder or even occult malignancy, is not the culprit. Diagnosis of disordered gastric motility involves pursuing the appropriate imaging study based on clinical suspicion. Once the diagnosis of a motility disorder is established, initial management is exclusively nonoperative and is usually successful. Operative intervention is reserved for the most severe and medically refractory cases.

Delayed Gastric Emptying

DGE is defined as abnormally slow gastric transit in the absence of physical obstruction. The estimated prevalence of DGE is 4% of the population, 80% of which are women.[20] The 3 most common causes, in descending order, are medications/drugs, diabetes, and postsurgical.[11] Medications and other drugs that commonly cause DGE are listed in **Box 1**.

The second most common cause of DGE is diabetes related. DGE can be found in 20% to 50% of diabetic patients,[21] and is usually associated with later stages of the disease. Although the pathophysiology of diabetic gastroparesis is not fully understood, there is certainly a multifactorial influence. Evidence suggests that both hyperglycemia and hyperinsulinemia suppress phase III of the MMC and result in an increase in pyloric contractility.[24] Both mechanisms contribute to DGE, as well as reduced gastric clearance in the fasting state with potential bezoar formation.[22,24] Hyperglycemia has also been shown to result in a direct myopathy of the gastric antrum.[22]

The third most common cause of DGE is postvagotomy gastroparesis. This disease entity encompasses vagotomy during an acid-reducing procedure, as well as inadvertent injury to the vagus or its gastric branches. Truncal vagotomy results in a 5% incidence of postoperative DGE, even when a concomitant drainage procedure is performed.[22] When performed correctly, highly selective vagotomy should not induce

Box 1
Medications and drugs that delay gastric emptying

Alcohol

Aluminum hydroxide antacids

Muscarinic cholinergic receptor antagonist

β-Agonists

Calcium channel blockers

Diphenhydramine

Glucagon

Dopamine agonists

Lithium

Ondansetron

Opioid analgesics

Phenothiazines

Tobacco/smoking

Tricyclic antidepressants

Data from Refs.[11,21–23]

DGE as the antral/pyloric innervation is left intact. Loss of vagal input eliminates a critical postprandial stimulus to the enteric nervous system, leading to reduced peristalsis of the distal stomach and resulting in DGE from a reduced ability to empty solids.[24] Vagotomy may also lead to loss of phase II of the MMC in the fasting state. Fortunately, fewer than 1% of these patients experience persistent, disabling symptoms.[24] Other causes of DGE are listed in **Box 2**. Of note, infections implicated in DGE include *Helicobacter pylori*, Epstein-Barr virus (EBV), and cytomegalovirus (CMV).[25] Fortunately, DGE from an infectious source is often self-limiting.[23]

Diagnosis

Patients with DGE often suffer from nausea, vomiting, bloating, early satiety, abdominal pain, and discomfort. These symptoms are made worse with the ingestion of meals proportionally higher in solid content.[22] Weight fluctuations are another common complaint. Although these symptoms are nonspecific, abdominal pain, bloating, and fullness best correlate with DGE.[28] Physical examination findings may include a rotund, tender, and possibly tympanic upper abdomen. Laboratory findings may show hypokalemia and a contraction alkalosis from poor intake and persistent vomiting.

The complex and often contradictory symptoms of DGE necessitate confirmatory imaging to establish a definitive diagnosis. The 4-hour radionucleotide colloid scintigraphy gastric emptying study (GES) is the gold standard for diagnosis.[7,29] This test can be performed using a radiolabeled liquid or solid meal, although the solid-based test is preferred because the liquid-based scan can be normal in advanced disease states.[20] The solid-meal GES is usually administered as an isotope-labeled, low-fat, scrambled-egg meal. Greater than 60% retention at 2 hours or greater than 10% retention at 4 hours confirms the diagnosis of DGE.[11,29]

Any suggestion of outlet obstruction should be initially ruled out with endoscopic evaluation. The presence of retained items in the stomach, especially phyto-bezoars,

Box 2
Causes of gastroparesis

Medications and other drugs (listed in Box 1)

Diabetes

Surgery-related, vagotomy, duodenectomy, postgastrectomy

Metabolic (hyperglycemia, hypokalemia, hypermagnesemia)

Hypopituitarism, hypoadrenalism, hypothyroidism

Chronic renal failure

Portal hypertension

Intra-abdominal malignancy

Infectious: *H pylori*, EBV, CMV

Autoimmune: Systemic sclerosis, systemic lupus erythematosus

Myotonic dystrophies

Central nervous system disorders (Parkinson disease, multiple sclerosis)

Peripheral nervous system disorders (amyloid neuropathy, Guillain-Barré, primary dysautonomia)

Psychiatric disorders (anorexia nervosa, rumination syndrome)

Data from Refs.[5,20,23,26,27]

indicates a high probability of DGE. A fluoroscopic GES can assess gastric emptying and evaluate potential outlet obstruction. Although not directly useful in the assessment of DGE, a barium upper GI series can be essential to rule out mechanical obstruction.[20] On very rare occasions, diagnostic laparotomy may be required to correctly distinguish a partial distal small bowel obstruction from a small bowel pseudo-obstruction with a component of DGE.[30]

Many other imaging modalities are available, each having inherent advantages and disadvantages. Real-time ultrasonography can be used to calculate gastric volumes after the ingestion of a liquid. Although this test is better for patients who should not be exposed to radiation, it is somewhat operator-dependent.[11,20,22] Contrasted MRI can be used with sequential axial scanning, and has the advantage of measuring multiple parameters simultaneously. Although supine positioning is an obvious disadvantage, this test has been found to correlate well with the gold standard scintigraphic GES.[11,20,22,31] Single-photon computed tomography can be obtained after intravenous administration of [^{99}Tc]pertechnetate. This isotope accumulates in the gastric wall and provides a 3-dimensional image of the stomach to measure real-time gastric volumes.[20,22]

Finally, patients can be given radiopaque markers to swallow. A follow-up abdominal radiograph obtained 6 hours after swallowing should demonstrate absence of markers from the stomach.[20] Although this test is simple and inexpensive, it cannot be directly correlated to the emptying of digestible material.[32]

Other options for assessment include the satiety test, which measures the amount of a liquid ingested until the patient reports feeling full. Although this parameter is reduced in DGE, the applicability of this test tends to be very subjective.[11,20,22] GI manometry uses an intraluminal catheter to measure gastric pressures in real time. A 4- to 5-hour fasting period is initially assessed, followed by a 2-hour postprandial period.[11,20,22] Manometry can help distinguish specific causes of DGE. For example, autonomic neuropathy would demonstrate normal fasting pattern due to inherent myogenic contraction, with the absence of conversion to the fed state. Conversely, DGE derived from a myopathy would demonstrate abnormal contractions of the gastric musculature.

Multiple other studies may have application in the assessment of DGE, but have not undergone full clinical validation. The barostat system uses a balloon in the stomach to measure pressure and volume.[20] This study has been shown to demonstrate gastric emptying effectively, but produces nonphysiologic gastric accommodation that limits its clinical usefulness.[31] An indirect assessment of gastric emptying using breath testing shows early promise. A ^{13}C-labeled substrate is ingested, which is metabolized in the intestine and eventually exhaled as $^{13}CO_2$. The rate of $^{13}CO_2$ exhalation is proportional to the gastric emptying rate.[11,20,22] Another method uses a radiotelemetry capsule, which constantly transmits a pH measurement. Gastric emptying time is the period from ingestion of the capsule until a neutral pH is obtained, signifying passage into the proximal duodenum.[20,22] This test has been shown to correlate with the findings of a simultaneously performed GES.[33]

Noninvasive techniques for measuring gastric motility in early stages of development show much promise for accurate assessment of the underlying electrical activity of the stomach. Electrogastrography (EGG) measures gastric potentials transcutaneously to assess for disordered motility. Tachygastria is defined as greater than 4 cycles per minute, and bradygastria is the presence of less than 2 cycles per minute.[11,20,22,34] While promising as a logical correlate to electrocardiography and the heart, cutaneous EGG cannot accurately predict the underlying abnormalities of gastric electrical activity and has been virtually abandoned by clinicians.

The inherent limitations of EGG have led to the development of magnetogastrography (MGG). MGG uses a superconducting magnetometer to measure surface current density of the magnetic fields overlying the abdominal wall generated by the electrical activity of the gastric smooth muscle. Because magnetic fields are not attenuated by the intervening tissues of the abdominal wall, a more accurate assessment of the underlying gastric electrical activity can be obtained. This information is translated to frequency, direction, amplitude, and velocity of the gastric slow wave. MGG shows great promise to accurately measure the underlying electromagnetic fields generated by the gastric smooth muscle.[35,36] Studies using this technology suggest that differences in the underlying gastric electrical activity can be linked to DGE (**Fig. 4**[36]).

Initial management

Initial management of DGE includes optimal medical therapy for any predisposing conditions (ie, glucose control in diabetics). Small, frequent meals are advocated to reduce symptoms. High-residue diets should also be avoided because of the risk of accumulation and bezoar formation.[37] Empiric acid-reducing therapy can be administered, but often will only treat concomitant gastroesophageal reflux without altering the underlying motility disorder.[4] Prokinetic and antiemetic medications are the mainstay of pharmacotherapy. Prokinetic agents include metoclopramide, erythromycin, and domperidone. Antiemetic agents include prochlorperazine, promethazine, and 5-hydroxytryptamine receptor agonist (ie, odansetron).[37] Other options include endoscopic intrapyloric botulinum toxin injection. Though purported to alleviate DGE caused by aberrant contractions at the gastric outlet, results have been disappointing.[4,37]

Surgical management

Operative management of DGE is reserved for severe and persistent symptoms refractory to medical management. Multiple options have been described, ranging from percutaneous gastrostomy to near total gastrectomy. Unfortunately, all traditional methods suffer from poor symptomatic relief and high recurrence rates, along with substantial morbidity associated with more drastic measures. A gastrostomy is an

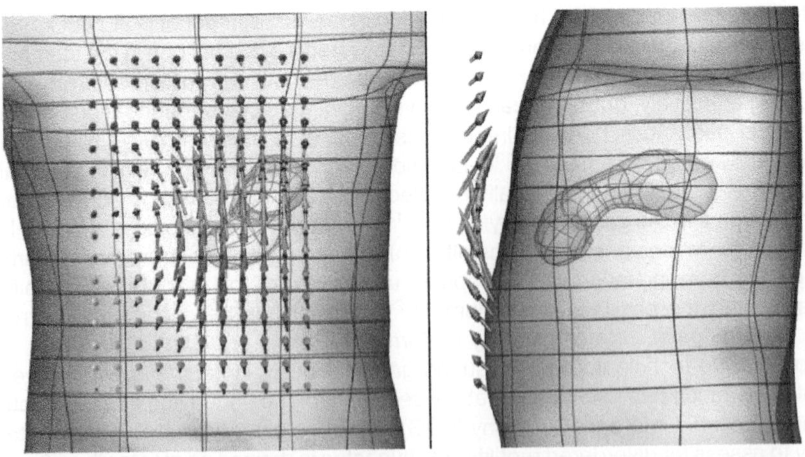

Fig. 4. Magnetogastrography (MGG). Illustration demonstrating a simulated surface current density recorded over the stomach by a superconducting magnetometer. (*From* Bradshaw L, Cheng L, Richards W, et al. Surface current density mapping for identification of gastric slow wave propagation. IEEE Trans Biomed Eng 2010. Available at: http://ieeexplore.ieee.org/lpdocs/epic03/wrapper.htm?arnumber=4895313; with permission.)

appealing option secondary to its relative ease of placement and low morbidity. A gastrostomy tube can be placed percutaneously with endoscopic or fluoroscopic assistance, or surgically via open or laparoscopic methods. A jejunostomy can be placed using all of these same methods, or via a new or previously placed gastrostomy.[38] Both function to provide enteral access for nutrition, which may be critical in cases of DGE resulting in severe malnutrition and weight loss. In these cases, enteral access is preferred over the multitude of complications arising from long-term intravenous nutrition.[4] Furthermore, a gastrostomy or jejunostomy also provides a mechanism to periodically release pressure from the upper GI tract to treat episodes of symptomatic distention resulting from gastroparesis.

The ultimate intervention for refractory DGE is subtotal or complete gastrectomy. This procedure should only be considered for the management of the most severe cases of DGE with no other alternative treatment.[39] While an extensive procedure in the best of circumstances, completion gastrectomy will often need to be performed in a poor surgical candidate with a history of systemic illness or multiple previous abdominal operations.[38] Reconstruction with a Roux-en-Y gastrojejunostomy is usually preferred. The best long-term improvements have been seen in patients undergoing completion gastrectomy for symptoms related to previous partial gastrectomy or vagotomy.[40–42]

Gastric neurostimulation

The overall poor results from conventional therapy, along with a greater understanding of gastric electrical physiology, have led to the development of gastric electrical stimulation devices. The first and only device to have received approval from the Food and Drug Administration (FDA) is the Enterra gastric neurostimulator (Medtronic, Minneapolis, MN). This device uses a low-energy, high-frequency (12 cycles per minute), and short-duration pulse to stimulate the gastric enteric nervous system.[37,43] During laparotomy or laparoscopy, paired electrodes are placed approximately 1 to 2 cm apart near the native pacing zone located on the greater curvature of the stomach.[37] These leads are tunneled to a pocket within the anterior abdominal wall containing the pulse generator.[37] Upper endoscopy can be considered after placement rule out any violation of the gastric lumen during placement.[44] Potential complications include pocket infection, erosion of the pulse generator, intestinal obstruction, and gastric lead breakage, dislodgment, or perforation.[37]

In a subjective study via questionnaire, Enterra therapy is consistently found to improve symptoms of DGE in over half of the patients studied, with more improvement reported in those patients suffering from diabetic than from idiopathic gastroparesis. Interestingly, these studies have also demonstrated that gastric neurostimulation can result in improvement in nausea and vomiting more readily than abdominal pain.[39,44] Indications for it use are also being expanded to post-operative DGE, with good preliminary results.[45] Improvements of these devices focus on less invasive placement techniques, using the same basic mechanism. Methods currently in development include cutaneous or percutaneous endoscopically placed electrodes.[46,47] A significant drawback of the Enterra neurostimulator is the lack of evidence to show that gastric emptying is altered in any way with this form of therapy.

A similar device, the Tantalus II (MetaCure, Kfar-Saba, Israel) system, is approved for use only in Europe, with current FDA approval for use within clinical trials. This device synchronizes to gastric slow waves and delivers electrical signals that serve to modulate gastric contractility. High-energy, low-frequency, and long-duration pulses stimulate the stomach at a rate slightly above the slow-wave rate of 3 cycles per minute. The device is placed in the same manner as the Enterra system, except

3 pairs of electrodes are placed in the gastric wall and are connected to the pulse generator. Lead pairs are placed at the fundus and the anterior and posterior antral wall, with each pair being placed 2 cm apart perpendicular to the long axis of the stomach.[48] Potential complications are also similar to those of the Enterra device. Unlike the Enterra device, Tantalus therapy has been found to pace the gastric musculature and accelerate gastric emptying of solids.[43,48] Of interest, the Tantalus system is also being explored as a treatment of type 2 diabetes mellitus via reduction in weight and blood glucose levels.[43]

Rapid Gastric Transit

Rapid gastric transit (RGT) describes a spectrum of symptoms resulting from accelerated flow of gastric contents into the small bowel.[49] The critical mechanism in this disorder is the transit of unprocessed or poorly processed hyperosmolar gastric contents into the proximal small bowel, not necessarily the speed of gastric emptying.[50] RGT can result from any functional impairment of the pyloric sphincter allowing hyperosmolar contents to abruptly enter the small bowel. RGT is best described by "dumping syndrome," the classically described postprandial symptoms following pyloroplasty or gastrectomy.

Dumping syndrome is categorized into two phases according to distinct symptoms. Early dumping occurs 15 to 30 minutes after eating when hyperosmolar luminal contents swiftly enter the proximal intestine; this leads to a sudden fluid shift into the intestine, resulting in nausea and vomiting, diarrhea, diaphoresis, hypotension, and possible syncope.[24] Furthermore, the hyperosmolar luminal contents trigger serotonin release from the argentaffin cells of the small intestine. Serotonin release results in massive peripheral and mesenteric vasodilation, further contributing to the hypotension-inducing fluid shifts of early-phase dumping.[51] Many other hormone levels are elevated in association with the dumping syndrome, including neurotensin, pancreatic polypeptide, enteroglucagon, peptide YY, insulin, glucagon, and glucagon-like peptide.[9,29,50] Late dumping, although variably present, results from the swift uptake of glucose and other sugars from the small bowel. This resultant hyperglycemia stimulates a reactive increase in insulin, along with rebound hypoglycemia and hypokalemia. The hypoglycemia that occurs with dumping typically manifests 45 to 60 minutes after the meal.

Etiology

Consequences of gastrectomy were traditionally the leading causes of RGT and dumping syndrome. Partial gastrectomy has been shown to result in dumping syndrome in 15% to 20% of cases, and in 6% to 14% of patients after truncal vagotomy and pyloroplasty.[29] Gastric resection with Roux-en-Y reconstruction results in some form of dumping symptoms in up to 70% of patients postoperatively, but most symptoms resolve with conservative intervention in the follow-up period.[29] This ability to recover normal function depends on the regeneration of the phase III MMC from within the jejunal limb.[52] Multiple procedures were devised to provide for the best functional results after gastrectomy. Pylorus-preserving gastrectomy has consistently been shown to provide the lowest incidence of dumping syndrome.[49] When resection of the distal stomach is required, distal gastrectomy with Roux-en-Y reconstruction has been shown to result in a reduced incidence of dumping syndrome as compared with Billroth I reconstruction.[49]

Anatomic alterations imposed by bariatric surgery constitute an increasing proportion of surgical causes of RGT. Symptomatic dumping syndrome was found in 0.3% of restrictive (decreased gastric capacity) procedures and 14.6% of combined restrictive and malabsorptive (decreased intestinal absorptive length) procedures.[53] Alternatively, vertical sleeve gastrectomy virtually eliminates any risk of postoperative dumping syndrome.[54–56] Other sources of RGT include any source of autonomic dysfunction, such as large-fiber neuropathy, neuropathy related to diabetes mellitus, amyloidosis, or idiopathic neuropathy.[19] Of interest, RGT occurs more often in early-stage diabetes than at any other time in the course of the disease.[57] Zollinger-Ellison syndrome and peptic ulcer disease are rare causes of RGT.[29]

Other rare causes of RGT include increased antral peristalsis or reduced pyloric resistance.[19] Furthermore, reduced gastric compliance can result in increased intragastric pressure and contributes to accelerated emptying. Causes of decreased compliance include gastric resection, vagotomy, post-fundoplication, or rumination syndrome.[1,4] Interruption of vagal efferents can lead to chronic gastric atony, with loss of receptive relaxation with increased intragastric pressure in response to a food bolus. This process results in bloating and early satiety with rapid emptying of liquids.[22] Tube feedings represent an iatrogenic source of RGT from reduced compliance, as the process of receptive relaxation initiated during swallowing is completely bypassed.

Diagnosis

Suspicion of RGT can be made on clinical grounds in patients demonstrating the aforementioned postprandial symptoms.[4] Formerly a barium GES was used to help confirm the diagnosis. A modified oral glucose challenge can also be employed, in which a 50-gram solution of glucose is administered the morning after a fast. Early evidence of a significant fluid shift (increased pulse rate >10 beats/min or hematocrit >3%) or late hypoglycemia (<60 mg/dL) confirms the diagnosis.[50] Alternatively, radionucleotide colloid scintigraphy using an isotope-labeled 2% scrambled-egg meal can be used, with a greater than 50% transit of luminal contents at 1 hour establishing the diagnosis.[29]

Initial management

Initial management of RGT includes dietary modification, minimizing liquids and any particularly hyperosmolar intake. Patients are encouraged to avoid liquids with or 2 hours after a meal. Small, high-protein, low-carbohydrate meals are encouraged, spreading out intake over 6 meals a day.[50] Lying down after meals can further help delay emptying time, as well as counteract any symptoms arising from hypovolemia.[50] The α-glucosidase inhibitor acarbose can be used to slow carbohydrate digestion and absorption, helping to prevent late reactive hyperglycemia.[4,50] Administration of the long-acting somatostatin analogue, octreotide acetate, has been shown to be highly effective in the treatment of medically refractory dumping syndrome. Octreotide functions by promoting the fasting state of intestinal motility along with inhibition of vasoactive hormone release.[4,9,50] One of the authors (W.O.R.) has successfully treated a small number of patients with severe dumping for over 10 years with small doses (10–50 μg subcutaneously) of octreotide acetate before meals.[9]

Surgical management

Operative intervention may be necessary for the most severe and refractory cases of RGT. Results from these "rescue operations" are unpredictable and often poor.[50] In addition, the morbidity of what is often a repeat operation must be considered. These facts emphasize attention to detail and patience during the initial trial of dietary modification and medical therapy, noting the success of the administration of octreotide acetate in severe cases.

The first surgical option is restoration of normal anatomy. Direct pyloric reconstruction may be of benefit for refractory RGT after vagotomy and pyroplasty.[50] In the few patients who develop disabling dumping syndrome after Roux-en-Y gastric bypass, failure of dietary and medical therapy to correct severe reactive hypoglycemia necessitates surgical revision to restore the original anatomy. The use of laparoscopy during reversal has been found to be feasible and safe.[58] Contraindications are previous vagotomy and pyloric obstruction.

A second surgical option includes the use of a reversed intestinal segment as a pyloric bypass.[24] This method, although effective, suffers from a high rate of obstruction necessitating yet another operative intervention. The third option for surgical management of RGT is modification of the anastomosis created during a previous gastric resection. Although a Billroth II construction could be converted to a Billroth I to take advantage of a lower rate of dumping syndrome, results have not shown particular success.[50] Roux-en-Y construction often leads to a delay in gastric emptying (Roux stasis syndrome), providing a versatile method for the treatment of RGE.[50,60] As with any Roux-en-Y bypass, the significant risk of marginal ulceration merits a concomitant vagotomy and hemigastrectomy.[59] A novel therapeutic approach involves the reduction of the diameter of the anastomotic channel to reduce gastric transit. Other methods currently in development and undergoing clinical validation include the endoscopic use of fibrin glue, suturing, and argon plasma coagulation.[61]

SUMMARY

Disordered gastric motility is primarily managed with dietary modification followed by appropriate pharmacotherapy. Traditional surgical interventions for the most severe cases tended to be formidable, rarely definitive, and fraught with complications. The increase in the number of bariatric procedures and predisposing conditions such as diabetes will continue to produce a significant number of these refractory cases. Improvements in minimally invasive procedures will provide options for earlier and more effective intervention, as well as opportunities for management in those formerly deemed poor surgical candidates.

REFERENCES

1. Wood JD. Neurogastroenterology and motility. In: Rhoades R, Bell DR, editors. Medical physiology: principles for clinical medicine. 3rd edition. Baltimore (MD): Lippincott Williams & Wilkins; 2008. p. 483–8.
2. Barrett KE. Gastric motility. In: Barrett KE, editor. Gastrointestinal physiology. Available at: http://www.accessmedicine.com/content.aspx?aID=2307328. Accessed June 22, 2011. [Chapter: 8].
3. Mercer DW, Liu TH, Castaneda A. Anatomy and physiology of the stomach. In: Yeo CJ, editor. Shackelford's surgery of the alimentary tract. 5th edition. Elsevier; 2002. p. 3.
4. Tack J. Gastric motor disorders. Best Pract Res Clin Gastroenterol 2007;21(4): 633–44.
5. Khoo J, Rayner CK, Feinle-Bisset C, et al. Gastrointestinal hormonal dysfunction in gastroparesis and functional dyspepsia. Neurogastroenterol Motil 2010;22(12): 1270–8.
6. Verkijk M, Gielkens HA, Lamers CB, et al. Effect of gastrin on antroduodenal motility: role of intraluminal acidity. Gastrointestin and Liver Physiol. Am J Physiol 1998;275(5):1209.

7. Kollmar O, Moussavian MR, Richter S, et al. Prophylactic octreotide and delayed gastric emptying after pancreaticoduodenectomy: results of a prospective randomized double-blinded placebo-controlled trial. Eur J Surg Oncol 2008; 34(8):868–75.
8. Richards WO, Geer R, O'Dorisio TM, et al. Octreotide acetate induces fasting small bowel motility in patients with dumping syndrome. J Surg Res 1990; 49(6):483–7.
9. Geer RJ, Richards WO, O'Dorisio TM, et al. Efficacy of octreotide acetate in treatment of severe postgastrectomy dumping syndrome. Ann Surg 1990;212(6):678–87.
10. Lu Y, Owyang C. Secretin-induced gastric relaxation is mediated by vasoactive intestinal polypeptide and prostaglandin pathways. Neurogastroenterol Motil 2009;21:754-e47.
11. Patrick A, Epstein O. Review article: gastroparesis. Aliment Pharmacol Ther 2008; 27(9):724–40.
12. Rees WD, Malagelada JR, Miller LJ, et al. Human interdigestive and postprandial gastrointestinal motor and gastrointestinal hormone patterns. Dig Dis Sci 1982; 27(4):321–9.
13. Hellström PM, Grybäck P, Jacobsson H. The physiology of gastric emptying. Best Pract Res Clin Anaesthesiol 2006;20(3):397–407.
14. Sun WM, Houghton LA, Read NW, et al. Effect of meal temperature on gastric emptying of liquids in man. Br Med J 1988;29(3):302.
15. Mishima Y, Amano Y, Takahashi Y, et al. Gastric emptying of liquid and solid meals at various temperatures. J Gastroenterol 2009;44(5):412–8.
16. Van Citters GW, Lin HC. The ileal brake: a fifteen-year progress report. Curr Gastroenterol Rep 1999;1(5):404–9.
17. Camilleri M. Functional dyspepsia: mechanisms of symptom generation and appropriate management of patients. Gastroenterol Clin North Am 2007;36(3):649–64.
18. Abell TL, Camilleri M, Donohoe K, et al. Consensus recommendations for gastric emptying scintigraphy: a joint report of the American Neurogastroenterology and Motility Society and the Society of Nuclear Medicine. J Nucl Med Technol 2008; 36(1):44–54.
19. Lawal A, Barboi A, Krasnow A, et al. Rapid gastric emptying is more common than gastroparesis in patients with autonomic dysfunction. Am J Gastroenterol 2007;102(3):618–23.
20. Waseem S, Moshiree B, Draganov PV. Gastroparesis: current diagnostic challenges and management considerations. World J Gastroenterol 2009;15(1):25.
21. Ajumobi AB, Griffin MB. Diabetic gastroparesis: evaluation and management. Hosp Physician 2008;44(3):27–35.
22. Hasler WL. Gastroparesis: symptoms, evaluation, and treatment. Gastroenterol Clin North Am 2007;36(3):619–47.
23. Thorn AR. Not just another case of nausea and vomiting: a review of postinfectious gastroparesis. J Am Acad Nurse Pract 2010;22(3):125–33.
24. Mercer DW, Robinson EK. Stomach. In: Townsend CM, Beauchamp RD, Evers BM, et al, editors. Sabiston textbook of surgery. 18th edition. Saunders; 2007. p. 1223–77. [Chapter: 47].
25. Naftali T, Yishai R, Zangen T, et al. Post-infectious gastroparesis: clinical and electerogastrographic aspects. J Gastroenterol Hepatol 2007;22(9):1423–8.
26. Golzarian J, Scott HW, Richards WO. Hypermagnesemia-induced paralytic ileus. Dig Dis Sci 1994;39(5):1138–42.
27. Lobrano A, Blanchard K, Abell TL, et al. Postinfectious gastroparesis related to autonomic failure: a case report. Neurogastroenterol Motil 2005;18:162–7.

28. Khayyam U, Sachdeva P, Gomez J, et al. Assessment of symptoms during gastric emptying scintigraphy to correlate symptoms to delayed gastric emptying. Neurogastroenterol Motil 2010;22(5):539–45.
29. Hejazi RA, Patil H, McCallum RW. Dumping syndrome: establishing criteria for diagnosis and identifying new etiologies. Dig Dis Sci 2009;55(1):117–23.
30. Richards WO, Williams LF. Pseudo-pseudo-obstruction. A clinically relevant concept. Am Surg 1989;55(1):26–31.
31. de Zwart IM, Haans JJ, Verbeek P, et al. Gastric accommodation and motility are influenced by the barostat device: assessment with magnetic resonance imaging. Am J Physiol Gastrointest Liver Physiol 2007;292(1):G208.
32. Camilleri M. Diabetic gastroparesis. N Engl J Med 2007;356(8):820.
33. Cassilly D, Kantor S, Knight LC, et al. Gastric emptying of a non-digestible solid: assessment with simultaneous SmartPill pH and pressure capsule, antroduodenal manometry, gastric emptying scintigraphy. Neurogastroenterol Motil 2008;20(4): 311–9.
34. Huerta-Franco R, Vargas-Luna M, Hernandez E, et al. Use of short-term bio-impedance for gastric motility assessment. Med Eng Phys 2009;31(7):770–4.
35. Bradshaw LA, Irimia A, Sims JA, et al. Biomagnetic signatures of uncoupled gastric musculature. Neurogastroenterol Motil 2009;21(7):778.
36. Bradshaw L, Cheng L, Richards W, et al. Surface current density mapping for identification of gastric slow wave propagation. IEEE Trans Biomed Eng 2009;56(8): 2131–9.
37. Friedenberg FK, Parkman HP. Management of delayed gastric emptying. Clin Gastroenterol Hepatol 2005;3:642–6.
38. Jones MP, Maganti K. A systematic review of surgical therapy for gastroparesis. Am J Gastroenterol 2003;98(10):2122–9.
39. Velanovich V. Quality of life and symptomatic response to gastric neurostimulation for gastroparesis. J Gastrointest Surg 2008;12(10):1656–63.
40. Eckhauser FE, Conrad M, Knol JA, et al. Safety and long-term durability of completion gastrectomy in 81 patients with postsurgical gastroparesis syndrome. Am Surg 1998;64(8):716–7.
41. Forstner-Barthell AW, Murr MM, Nitecki S, et al. Near-total completion gastrectomy for severe postvagotomy gastric stasis: analysis of early and long-term results in 62 patients. J Gastrointest Surg 1999;3(1):15–23.
42. Speicher JE, Thirlby RC, Burggraaf J, et al. Results of completion gastrectomies in 44 patients with postsurgical gastric atony. J Gastrointest Surg 2009;13(5): 874–80.
43. Maranki J, Parkman HP. Gastric electric stimulation for the treatment of gastroparesis. Curr Gastroenterol Rep 2007;9(4):286–94.
44. Maranki JL, Lytes V, Meilahn JE, et al. Predictive factors for clinical improvement with Enterra gastric electric stimulation treatment for refractory gastroparesis. Dig Dis Sci 2007;53(8):2072–8.
45. Salameh JR, Schmieg RE, Runnels JM, et al. Refractory gastroparesis after Roux-en-Y gastric bypass: surgical treatment with implantable pacemaker. J Gastrointest Surg 2007;11(12):1669–72.
46. Sallam HS, Chen JD, Pasricha PJ. Feasibility of gastric electric stimulation by percutaneous endoscopic transgastric electrodes. Gastrointest Endosc 2008; 68(4):754–9.
47. Wang J, Song J, Hou X, et al. Effects of cutaneous gastric electrical stimulation on gastric emptying and postprandial satiety and fullness in lean and obese subjects. J Clin Gastroenterol 2010;44(5):335.

48. Sanmiguel CP, Haddad W, Aviv R, et al. The TANTALUS system for obesity: effect on gastric emptying of solids and ghrelin plasma levels. Obes Surg 2007;17(11):1503–9.
49. Mine S, Sano T, Tsutsumi K, et al. Large-scale investigation into dumping syndrome after gastrectomy for gastric cancer. J Am Coll Surg 2010;211:628–36.
50. Tack J, Arts J, Caenepeel P, et al. Pathophysiology, diagnosis and management of postoperative dumping syndrome. Nat Rev Gastroenterol Hepatol 2009;6(10): 583–90.
51. Deitel M. The change in the dumping syndrome concept. Obes Surg 2008; 18(12):1622–4.
52. Tomita R, Fujisaki S, Tanjoh K, et al. Studies on gastrointestinal hormone and jejunal interdigestive migrating motor complex in patients with or without early dumping syndrome after total gastrectomy with Roux-en-Y reconstruction for early gastric cancer. Am J Surg 2003;185(4):354–9.
53. Monteforte MJ, Turkelson CM. Bariatric surgery for morbid obesity. Obes Surg 2000;10(5):391–401.
54. Iannelli A, Anty R, Schneck AS, et al. Inflammation, insulin resistance, lipid disturbances, anthropometrics, and metabolic syndrome in morbidly obese patients: a case control study comparing laparoscopic Roux-en-Y gastric bypass and laparoscopic sleeve gastrectomy. Surgery 2011;149(3):364–70.
55. Peterli R, Wölnerhanssen B, Peters T, et al. Improvement in glucose metabolism after bariatric surgery: comparison of laparoscopic Roux-en-Y gastric bypass and laparoscopic sleeve gastrectomy: a prospective randomized trial. Ann Surg 2009;250(2):234.
56. Fuks D, Verhaeghe P, Brehant O, et al. Results of laparoscopic sleeve gastrectomy: a prospective study in 135 patients with morbid obesity. Surgery 2009; 145(1):106–13.
57. Ariga H, Imai K, Chen C, et al. Does ghrelin explain accelerated gastric emptying in the early stages of diabetes mellitus? Am J Physiol Regul Integr Comp Physiol 2008;294(6):R1807.
58. Dapri G, Cadière GB, Himpens J. Laparoscopic reconversion of Roux-en-Y gastric bypass to original anatomy: technique and preliminary outcomes. Obes Surg 2010. DOI:10.1007/s11695-010-0252-6.
59. Dempsey DT. Stomach. In: Brunicardi FC, Andersen DK, Billiar TR, et al, editors. Schwartz's Principles of Surgery, 9th edition. Available at: http://www.accessmedicine.com/content.aspx?aID=5030324. Accessed June 22, 2011. [Chapter: 26].
60. Hoya Y, Mitsumori N, Yanaga K. The advantages and disadvantages of a Roux-en-Y reconstruction after a distal gastrectomy for gastric cancer. Surg Today 2009;39(8):647–51.
61. Fernández-Esparrach G, Lautz DB, Thompson CC. Peroral endoscopic anastomotic reduction improves intractable dumping syndrome in Roux-en-Y gastric bypass patients. Surg Obes Relat Dis 2010;6(1):36–40.

Emergency Ulcer Surgery

Constance W. Lee, MD[a], George A. Sarosi Jr, MD[a,b,*]

KEYWORDS

• Peptic ulcer • Bleeding • Perforation • Surgery • Management

Once one of the most common indications for gastric surgery, the rate of elective surgery for peptic ulcer disease has been declining steadily over the past 3 decades. Data from American surgical training programs and Scandinavian national audits have shown a decrease in the rate of elective ulcer surgery of between 80% and 97% during the 1980s and 1990s.[1,2] During this same time period, the rate of emergency ulcer surgery rose by 44%. In the United States in 2006, roughly 25,000 operations were performed for bleeding or perforated peptic ulcers.[3] These time trends mean that the gastrointestinal surgeon is likely to be called on to manage the emergent complications of peptic ulcer disease in an elderly and ill patient without substantial experience in elective peptic ulcer disease surgery.[4] The goal of this review is to familiarize surgeons with our evolving understanding of the pathogenesis, epidemiology, presentation, and management of peptic ulcer disease in the emergency setting, with a focus on peptic ulcer disease–associated bleeding and perforation.

PATHOGENESIS OF PEPTIC ULCER DISEASE

The classic understanding of the pathogenesis of peptic ulcer disease is that it represents an imbalance between the toxicity of the gastric injurious forces of acid and pepsin and the mucosal defense mechanisms of the stomach and duodenum. Classically, the dictum was "no acid, no ulcer," as most ulcers were thought to be a consequence of excessive acid secretion caused by smoking, alcohol use, stress, or other environmental factors.[5] In this model, the pathogenesis was multifactorial, and many of the underlying factors were difficult to modify. Treatment of peptic ulcer disease needed to be chronic and was directed at the reduction of acid secretion either by vagotomy and/or surgical elimination of acid-secreting gastric mucosa or by chronic use of medications such as H2 antagonists or proton pump inhibitors (PPI).

The authors have nothing to disclose.

[a] Department of Surgery, University of Florida College of Medicine, 1600 Southwest Archer Road, PO Box 100109, Gainesville, FL 32610-0109, USA

[b] NF/SG VA Medical Center, 1601 SW Archer Road, Gainesville, FL 32608, USA

* Corresponding author. Department of Surgery, University of Florida College of Medicine, 1600 Southwest Archer Road, PO Box 100109, Gainesville, FL 32610-0109.

E-mail address: george.sarosi@surgery.ufl.edu

Surg Clin N Am 91 (2011) 1001–1013
doi:10.1016/j.suc.2011.06.008
0039-6109/11/$ – see front matter. Published by Elsevier Inc.

Our understanding of peptic ulcer pathogenesis was revolutionized by the discovery of the presence of the bacterium *Helicobactor pylori* in association with most gastric and duodenal ulcers in the early 1980s.[6] Over the next 10 years, multiple trials demonstrated that effective eradication of *H pylori* with a short course of antibiotics and PPIs resulted in relapse-free cure of the vast majority of ulcers. This led to a National Institutes of Health consensus conference in 1994 that recommended treatment of *H pylori* as the primary target of ulcer treatment.[7] With our increased understanding of the biology of *H pylori*, it is now clear that infection of the gastric mucosa with *H pylori* is responsible for most of the observed changes in gastric acid secretion observed in peptic ulcers. Patients with predominantly antral infection have impaired negative feedback of acid secretion, resulting in increased gastric acid production, and they develop duodenal and pre-pyloric ulcers. Patients with uniform infection throughout the stomach often have low acid production secondary to inflammation of the gastric body, which impairs the normal function of the acid-secreting mucosa and they frequently develop gastric ulcers. The effects of *H pylori* infection on acid secretion are beautifully described in a recent review, and nicely explain the observed clinical finding of differential acid secretion in duodenal and gastric ulcers.[5]

The use of aspirin and nonsteroidal anti-inflammatory drugs (NSAIDs) has long been recognized as an important case of peptic ulcer disease. These drugs inhibit the production of prostaglandins in the stomach that play a critical role in the mucosal defenses of the stomach against acid-induced and pepsin-induced injury.[8] In the stomach, prostaglandins stimulate mucus and bicarbonate production, and play an important role in the regulation of gastric mucosal blood flow. By inhibiting mucosal defense mechanisms against acid-mediated injury, NSAIDs are able to cause peptic ulceration independently, but also synergize with *H pylori* infection to cause peptic ulcers.[9] Our current understanding of peptic ulcer disease suggests that *H pylori* and NSAID use, either alone or in combination, are the causative agents for the vast majority of peptic ulcers. This new understanding of peptic ulcer disease implies that the great majority of peptic ulcer disease is the result of treatable or modifiable causes. Based on this understanding of the pathogenesis of peptic ulcer disease, the classic surgical approach directed at reducing acid production must be carefully reevaluated.

THE EPIDEMIOLOGY OF PEPTIC ULCER DISEASE

Once relatively common across all age groups, in the 21st century peptic ulcer disease is predominantly a disease of the elderly. Patients presenting with complications of peptic ulcer disease are most commonly in the seventh and eighth decades of life and there is a male predominance, with roughly 1.5 times as many cases in men than women.[3,10] Overall, there has been a marked decline in the incidence of all peptic ulcer disease, with data from multiple countries showing declines in ulcer hospitalization rates of 40% to 50% over the past 3 decades.[1,3,11] Duodenal ulcer is more common than gastric ulcer, although the largest decreases in ulcer incidence have been seen in duodenal ulcer.[10] Despite a declining incidence overall of peptic ulcer disease, the incidence of peptic ulcer disease complicated by either bleeding or perforation has remained constant or in fact even increased. Although the data are inconsistent in different countries, data from Finland and the Netherlands suggest that the rate of ulcer complications and the need for emergent ulcer surgery may have increased slightly over the past 30 years.[1,11]

These epidemiologic changes make sense with our new understanding of the pathophysiology of peptic ulcers. The rate of *H pylori* infection has been decreasing over time, both as a consequence of improved sanitation, treatment of infection, and a cohort effect. This likely explains the decrease overall in ulcer disease and aging of the ulcer patient. At the same time, with an aging population and increased use of NSAIDs, the reasons for increase in ulcer complications particularly in elderly individuals seems clear. For the surgeon dealing with patients with ulcer emergencies, this means increasingly being called on to offer surgical therapy to elderly frail patients.

BLEEDING PEPTIC ULCER

Presentation and Initial Management

Patients with bleeding from peptic ulcer will usually present with hematemesis, melena, or both. In the cases of massive bleeding, they can occasionally present with hematochezia. Many patients will present with hemodynamic findings of significant volume loss or even shock. Patients may also report a history of syncope before presentation, which should suggest significant blood loss. The initial management of all nonvariceal upper gastrointestinal (GI) bleeding is directed at obtaining intravenous access, ensuring the availability of blood for possible transfusion, and initiating resuscitation of the patient with either crystalloid solutions or blood if evidence of significant blood loss exists. The primary therapeutic goal in a patient with acute upper GI bleeding is control of bleeding, and the goal of a surgeon in managing a bleeding peptic ulcer is to provide definitive hemostasis. The challenge in managing bleeding peptic ulcers is that many patients will stop bleeding spontaneously, and only 5% to 10% of patients with bleeding ulcers will require surgery. To help identify patients likely to require intervention for bleeding control, and those at high risk for rebleeding and death from bleeding ulcers, several scoring systems based on clinical and endoscopic variables have been developed. The use of the prognostic systems for risk stratification is one of the major recommendations of a recently published international consensus statement on upper GI bleeding, and surgeons managing peptic ulcers should be familiar with their use.[12] The Blatchford score uses clinical and laboratory data, such as hemodynamic parameters; hemoglobin; and blood, urea, nitrogen level; and comorbid conditions to assess patients and can accurately identify patients at low risk of requiring intervention. The full scoring system is outlined in **Table 1**. Based on the Blatchford initial data, patients with a score of 3 or lower have a less than 6% chance of requiring intervention for hemostasis, whereas those with a score of 6 or higher have a greater than 50% chance of requiring intervention for control of bleeding.[13]

Endoscopic Intervention

The most important step in the management of a patient with a bleeding peptic ulcer is to arrange for urgent upper GI endoscopy. Upper GI endoscopy is critical in establishing the etiology of the bleeding, of which up to 60% is related to peptic ulcer disease.[14] More importantly, in most cases of active GI bleeding, endoscopic hemostatic techniques will be successful in controlling the source of bleeding. Meta-analysis of data in the early 1990s demonstrated that endoscopic therapy is effective at controlling peptic ulcer bleeding and reducing the risk of mortality and the need for surgical intervention.[15,16] More recent data have shown that the use of epinephrine injection combined with an additional technique, such as thermal contact, sclerosant, or clipping improves success in controlling initial bleeding.[17] In the hands of a skilled endoscopist, bleeding can initially be controlled in almost all cases. Essentially all patients with bleeding peptic ulcers should undergo upper endoscopy before the consideration of surgical therapy. It is important, however, for the surgeon to be present at

Table 1
Blatchford score

Blood urea nitrogen (BUN mg/dL)	
18.2–22.4	2
22.4–28	3
28–70	4
>70	6
Hemoglobin for men (g/dL)	
12–13	1
10–12	3
<10	6
Hemoglobin for women (g/dL)	
10–12	1
< 10	6
Systolic blood pressure mm Hg	
100–109	1
90–99	2
<90	3
Heart rate >100 bpm	1
Presentation with melena	1
Presentation with syncope	2
Hepatic disease	2
History of heart failure	2

Adapted from Blatchford O, Murray WR, Blatchford M. A risk score to predict need for treatment for upper-gastrointestinal haemorrhage. Lancet 2000;356(9238):1318–21.

the time of endoscopy, as important anatomic information will be gained during the endoscopic procedure. Failure of initial endoscopic hemostasis attempts is one of the indications for surgery in bleeding peptic ulcers.

Despite the high success rates of initial endoscopic hemostasis, roughly 15% to 20% of patients will experience re-bleeding from their ulcer. Rockall and colleagues[18] identified in 1996 that re-bleeding in patients with peptic ulcer disease is an important contributor to mortality risk. Based on a large cohort of patients, they devised a clinical scoring system based on patient characteristics and endoscopic findings that could be used to predict mortality and risk of re-bleeding in patients with peptic ulcer disease. Patients with a Rockall score of 3 or lower have a risk of re-bleeding of 11% and a mortality rate of less than 5%, whereas those with a score of 5 or higher have a re-bleeding rate of 25% and a greater than 10% risk of death. The components of the Rockall score are summarized in **Table 2**. Further study of the Rockall score has suggested that it is better at predicting mortality than re-bleeding, and has led to multiple attempts to better define the risk factors for re-bleeding. In a recent systematic review, 6 factors were identified as independent predictors of re-bleeding: hemodynamic instability, comorbid illnesses, active bleeding at endoscopy, ulcer size larger than 2 cm, and ulcer location in either the posterior duodenum or lesser curvature of the stomach.[19]

The role of the surgeon in patients at risk for re-bleeding after endoscopic hemostasis remains an area of controversy. Data from the 1980s, before widespread availability of modern endoscopic techniques for hemostasis, could not prove that early

Table 2
Rockall score

Variable	0	1	2	3
Age	<60	60–79	≥80	—
Shock	No shock	Tachycardia	Hypotension	
Comorbidity	None		Cardiac disease	Liver or kidney failure
Diagnosis	Mallory-Weiss or no diagnosis	All other diagnoses	Upper GI malignancy	
Stigmata of recent hemorrhage	None or dark spot		Blood in GI tract, bleeding or visible vessel, adherent clot	

Abbreviation: GI, gastrointestinal.

Adapted from Rockall TA, Logan RF, Devlin HB, et al. Risk assessment after acute upper gastrointestinal haemorrhage. Gut 1996;38(3):316–21.

operation for ulcers without active bleeding improved mortality, but it did show that it resulted in an increase in the number of patients undergoing operation.[20,21] One small trial using modern endoscopic hemostasis techniques compared early elective operation with endoscopic retreatment per protocol after initial endoscopic control of ulcer bleeding. This trial showed that patients who underwent early elective surgery were less likely to re-bleed, but showed no difference in overall mortality or need for emergency surgery.[22] It is worth noting that more than 75% of the patients receiving endoscopic therapy achieved definitive hemostasis without surgery. These data agree with the results of an elegant randomized controlled trial performed by Lau and colleagues,[23] which demonstrated that endoscopic retreatment of peptic ulcers that re-bled after initial endoscopic treatment was successful in nearly 75% of patients and associated with similar mortality and significantly fewer complications than immediate surgery for re-bleeding. In this study, 2 factors predicted failure of endoscopic retreatment for recurrent bleeding: an ulcer larger than 2 cm and patients who developed hypotension with the recurrent bleeding. Taken altogether, these studies suggest that early elective surgery for bleeding peptic ulcer does not reduce the mortality risk, but it does reduce the risk of re-bleeding. It seems reasonable to consider early elective operative intervention in those patients who are at high risk of recurrent bleeding, such as those with ulcers larger than 2 cm, hypotension on presentation, or with posterior duodenal or lesser curvature gastric ulcers. This recommendation must be balanced against significant risk of complications and death in this elderly frail patient population, and requires the exercise of careful surgical judgment.

Operative Approach

The primary goal of any operation for a bleeding peptic ulcer is hemorrhage control. Classically, the secondary goal of surgery was treatment of the underlying ulcer diathesis. With our current understanding of the underlying causes of peptic ulcers and the advent of potent acid-suppressive medications, the need for surgical reduction of acid secretion is less clear. The preferred operative approach to a peptic ulcer will depend on the location of the ulcer, and for this reason it is important for the surgeon caring for the patient to be present during upper GI endoscopy to obtain precise information on the location of the ulcer.

Bleeding gastric ulcers are generally best treated by excision of the ulcer and repair of the resulting gastric defect. Excision or biopsy of the ulcer is important, as 4% to 5% of benign-appearing ulcers are actually malignant ulcers.[24] For ulcers along the greater curvature of the stomach, antrum, or body of the stomach, wedge excision of the ulcer and closure of the resulting defect can easily be achieved in most cases without causing significant deformation of the stomach. Gastric ulcers along the lesser curvature of the stomach are more problematic. Because of the rich arcade of vessels from the left gastric artery, wedge excision of these ulcers is more difficult than in other locations, and the subsequent closure of the gastric defect is much more likely to result in deformation of the stomach and ether luminal obstruction or gastric volvulus of the resulting J-shaped stomach. For distal gastric ulcers along the lesser curvature in the area of the incisura angularis, a distal gastrectomy with either a Bilroth I or Bilroth II reconstruction is often the easiest method of excising the ulcer and restoring GI continuity. A special case is the proximal gastric ulcer near the gastroesophageal (GE) junction. Wedge excision of these ulcers will often result in compromise of the GE junction and leak. In most patients, the easiest approach is an anterior gastrotomy with biopsy and oversewing of the ulcer from inside the gastric lumen. With this approach, it is relatively easy to avoid compromising the GE junction. In the event that ulcer excision is necessary, a Csendes procedure, a distal gastrectomy with tongue-shaped extension of the lesser curve resection margin to include the ulcer and subsequent Roux-en-Y esophagogastrojejunostomy, is an excellent option.[25]

The standard approach to a bleeding duodenal ulcer is to perform an anterior longitudinal duodenotomy extending across the pylorus to the distal stomach. The bleeding vessel, often the gastroduodenal artery, is ligated in the ulcer crater by placing a figure of 8 suture at the top and the bottom of the ulcer crater to control the artery proximally and distally. A third suture is placed as a U-stitch underneath the ulcer to control the transverse pancreatic branches that enter the gastroduodenal artery posteriorly. The transverse duodenal incision is then closed vertically to construct a Heineke-Mikulicz pyloroplasty. Classically a truncal vagotomy is then performed to reduce the risk of recurrent ulceration. The role of the vagotomy in 2011 is unclear. Our modern understanding of the pathogenesis of peptic ulcer suggests that treatment of *H pylori* and elimination of NSAID use should result in cure of the underlying risk of ulcer. Further, with the advent of PPIs it is now possible to medically eliminate gastric acid production without the side effects of vagotomy. Although level 1 data exist for perforated duodenal ulcer, demonstrating that *H pylori* treatment eliminates the need for definitive ulcer surgery, there is to date no trial that confirms this finding in the case of bleeding duodenal ulcer.[26] Despite the lack of level 1 evidence, surveys of surgeons in the United Kingdom[27] and national data from the United States[3] suggest that most surgeons no longer perform a vagotomy as a component of operation for bleeding duodenal ulcer.

Although duodenotomy with direct control of the bleeding site with or without vagotomy is the most commonly used approach for a bleeding duodenal ulcer, there are some data to suggest that a more extensive operation may be associated with a lower re-bleeding rate. In 1993, Millat and colleagues[28] published a randomized controlled trial comparing vagotomy and pyloroplasty with gastric resection combined with ulcer excision. The found that the re-bleeding rate was higher (17% vs 3%) with vagotomy and pyloroplasty, but the overall mortality was not different. The major complication rate, mostly duodenal leaks, was significantly higher after gastric resection. An important caveat to these data is that this study was performed before widespread use of PPIs and *H pylori* treatment, and it is unclear that there is still a place for aggressive surgical treatment of the underlying ulcer disease now that medical therapy has replaced surgical therapy as the mainstay of ulcer treatment. In patients without significant comorbidities, who are not in shock at the time of operation, a more aggressive surgical approach may be warranted in patients with large posterior duodenal ulcers. Given the challenges of dealing with the difficult duodenal stump in a large posterior duodenal ulcer, this approach should be undertaken only by surgeons with significant experience in ulcer surgery.

Despite the best surgical efforts, re-bleeding after vagotomy and pyloroplasty occurs in between 6% and 17% of cases.[28,29] Endoscopic therapy is generally not an option after a recent duodenotomy, leaving 2 options: either reoperation or transcatheter arterial embolization (TAE). Classically, reoperation was the procedure of choice for re-bleeding after duodenotomy. In the case of reoperation for recurrent bleeding, most surgeons have advocated a more extensive operation, usually distal gastrectomy with or without vagotomy and ulcer excision or exclusion. This approach is unfortunately fraught with complications and associated with high operative mortality.[28,29] More recently, several investigators have advocated TAE as a viable alternative to operative treatment for ulcer bleeding refractory to endoscopy. Without a head-to-head trial, it is unclear whether TAE should replace surgery as a primary approach to bleeding control, but data from 2 large series suggest that TAE can achieve long-term hemostasis in roughly 75% of patients with recurrent bleeding after duodenotomy and ulcer oversewing.[30,31] Given the significant risk of complication or mortality in reoperation for recurrent bleeding, TAE, when available, should be the first-line therapy for recurrent bleeding after duodenotomy and ulcer oversewing.

PERFORATED ULCER

The therapeutic goal in a perforated peptic ulcer is to repair the hole in the GI tract and treat peritoneal contamination. Unlike in the case of bleeding duodenal ulcers, surgery is the mainstay of treatment for perforated peptic ulcers. Most perforated ulcers occur in the duodenum and pyloric channel. In an analysis of 40 trials of perforated peptic ulcer disease, perforation was most common at the duodenal bulb (62%), followed by the pyloric region (20%) and the gastric body (18%).[32] Although most patients who present with ulcer perforation have no prior history of ulcer disease, risk factors for perforation include the prior history of ulcer disease or use of NSAIDs.[33] In patients on NSAID therapy, there is a greater risk of ulcer perforation with a history of prior ulcer, age older than 60 years, concomitant use of alendronate, selective serotonin reuptake inhibitors, steroids, or anticoagulants.[34–37]

Presentation

Classically, the presentation of a perforated peptic ulcer is described as a 3-stage process.[38] Initial symptoms, occurring within 2 hours of perforation, include the abrupt onset of abdominal pain. The pain may initially be focused at the epigastrum, but it can quickly become generalized. Between 2 and 12 hours of perforation, the abdominal pain worsens and there may be significant pain with palpation of the hypogastrum and right lower quadrant secondary to drainage of succus from the perforation. Twelve hours after perforation, in addition to increasing pain, the patient may have fever, signs of hypovolemia, and abdominal distention.

Evaluation

It is important to quickly diagnose a perforated peptic ulcer. The prognosis is improved if treatment is provided within 6 hours of perforation, whereas a delay in treatment beyond 12 hours following perforation is associated with an increase in both morbidity and mortality.[38,39] In a prospective study of patients with duodenal ulcer perforations, Boey and colleagues[40] identified that perforations older than 48 hours, preoperative shock, and concurrent medical illness were associated with an increase in mortality.

In a patient with an appropriate history, if free air is present on an upright chest or abdominal x-ray or computed tomography (CT) scan, no additional testing is required before proceeding with treatment. However, direct findings of perforation are not identified in 10% to 20% of patients with a perforated duodenal ulcer.[41] An upper GI study or abdominal CT scan with oral contrast may be performed to confirm the diagnosis.

The patient should be evaluated for *H pylori* infection, as knowledge of a patient's *H pylori* status can play an important role in treatment decisions. *H pylori* infection is present in 70% to 90% of duodenal ulcers and 30% to 60% of gastric ulcers, and antibiotic therapy is very effective at eradication.[42] Noninvasive testing options include urea breath testing, stool antigen testing, and serology. Stool antigen testing is a modern and rapid method of gaining information on a patient's *H pylori* status in the preoperative period. A monoclonal stool antigen test has a 94% sensitivity, 97% specificity, and is processed in an hour.[43] A rapid stool antigen test may be processed within 5 minutes; however, the sensitivity is 76% and specificity 98%.[44]

Treatment

Medical management of a perforated peptic ulcer consists of fluid resuscitation, nasogastric decompression, acid suppression, and empiric antibiotic therapy. Antibiotic therapy should cover enteric gram-negative rods, anaerobes, oral flora, and fungus.[45,46] A nonsurgical treatment plan consisting of only the aforementioned medical management has been proposed for patients with contained perforation at high risk for operative complications.[47] Despite the appeal of nonoperative therapy in high-risk patients, the application of this strategy is likely limited, as was demonstrated in a randomized, controlled trial of nonoperative treatment for perforated peptic ulcers in which patients older than 70 years were less likely to improve with conservative management.[48]

Operative intervention is almost always indicated in the treatment of perforated peptic ulcers. Unfortunately, emergency surgery for a perforated peptic ulcer has a 6% to 30% risk of mortality.[39] In the setting of emergency surgery for perforated peptic ulcer, several variables have been independently associated with an increased risk of mortality, including age, American Society of Anesthesiologists (ASA) class, shock on admission, hypoalbuminemia on admission, an elevated serum creatinine, and preoperative metabolic acidosis.[49] Unfortunately, most of these adverse prognostic factors are not modifiable, and despite substantial advances in medical care, there has been little change in the mortality of perforated ulcer over the past 15 years.[3]

The choice of operation will depend on the site of perforation found at exploration. Duodenal and pyloric channel perforations are the most common sites of ulcer perforation and are functionally grouped as duodenal perforations. The most common technique for the management of a perforated duodenal ulcer is a patch repair with an omental pedicle, commonly referred to as a Graham patch or omentopexy.[50] In this technique, the ulcer is not closed, but instead a pedicle of vascularized omentum is sutured over the perforation site with multiple interrupted sutures. These repairs may be performed by a laparoscopic or open approach, but ulcers larger than 10 mm appear to increase the risk of conversion to open surgery. In a randomized controlled trial of 121 patients with perforated peptic ulcer disease, Siu and colleagues[51] demonstrated significantly lower analgesic requirements, postoperative hospital length of stay, and time away from work in patients receiving a laparoscopic repair. Importantly, there were no significant differences between the groups receiving an open or laparoscopic repair in terms of mortality, incidence of reoperation, or in the identification of postoperative intra-abdominal fluid collections. Classically repair of a perforated duodenal ulcer was accompanied by a definitive ulcer operation, either a vagotomy and pyloroplasty or a patch repair and a parietal cell vagotomy. However, with our improved understanding of the pathogenesis of peptic ulcers, it appears that definitive ulcer surgery is no longer necessary in most cases. Patch repair of the perforation with concomitant medical therapy is often sufficient for patients with ulcer disease secondary to *H pylori* infection or NSAIDs. A randomized study of 99 patients with perforated duodenal ulcers infected with *H pylori* treated with a patch repair demonstrated that successful treatment of *H pylori* significantly decreased ulcer recurrence from 38% to 5%, leading the investigators to conclude that a definitive ulcer procedure is not necessary in this setting.[26] In light of these data, knowledge of a patient's *H pylori* status before surgery cannot be understated.

In the rare patient with a history of *H pylori*–negative peptic ulcer disease or those who are unable to stop NSAID therapy, a definitive ulcer procedure may be performed if the patient is hemodynamically stable and has minimal intra-abdominal contamination. In this setting, a truncal vagotomy and pyloroplasty, omental patch and parietal cell vagotomy, or an antrectomy with truncal vagotomy have all been advocated as suitable repairs. Vagotomy and pyloroplasty is the easiest operation to perform, but has a 10% to 15% ulcer recurrence rate and exposes the patient to all of the complications of dumping and post-vagotomy syndromes. Omental patch with parietal cell vagotomy avoids most of the complications of dumping and post-vagotomy syndrome, but is a more challenging operation and high ulcer recurrence rates have been reported in inexperienced hands.[52] The benefits of a vagotomy with antrectomy are that the procedure may be applied to a variety of situations, and that the ulcer recurrence rate is very low. The disadvantages are that the operative mortality is higher than either of the other procedures, and the surgeon is forced to deal with an often chronically scarred duodenal stump and the complications of duodenal stump leak or anastomotic failure. The choice of definitive operation should depend on the experience of the surgeon, but in the absence of significant experience with ulcer surgery, vagotomy and pyloroplasty or not performing definitive surgery in the emergent setting seems prudent.

In the case of a perforated gastric ulcer, either ulcer excision and repair of the defect or biopsy and omental patch are the most expeditious approach in the emergency setting. Because malignancy has been reported in 4% to 14% of gastric perforations, biopsy or excision of the ulcer when feasible is important.[53] For a gastric ulcer located along the greater curvature, antrum, or body of the stomach, simple wedge excision of the ulcer is easy to perform, often with a single fire of a linear stapler, simultaneously obtaining tissue for biopsy and closing the perforation. Although no trials have been conducted comparing the techniques, this could be performed with either an open or laparoscopic approach. As with bleeding ulcers, ulcers along the lesser curvature of the stomach are more challenging because of the left gastric artery arcade, and the GE junction in high lesser curve ulcers. For distal lesser curve ulcers, distal gastrectomy can be performed with similar mortality to that seen with patch or simple excision.[54] The operative approach to perforation of an ulcer located next to the esophagogastric junction may include a subtotal gastrectomy to include the ulcer with a Roux-en-Y esophagogastrojejunostomy as described previously for bleeding ulcers.

A particularly challenging clinical scenario is the perforated giant duodenal ulcer. With a duodenal ulcer perforation larger than 2 cm, there is an increased risk of repair failure with omental patch repair, with leak rates of up to 12% reported.[55] In the setting of a giant perforated duodenal ulcer, there is no standard management. Recommendations for repair include omental patch, controlled tube duodenostomy, jejunal pedicled graft, jejunal serosal patch, pedicled omental plug, partial gastrectomy, and gastric disconnection.[55–57] The pedicled omental plug is an intriguing and easy option for this problem. In this procedure, an nasogastric (NG) tube is passed out through the perforation and a tongue of omentum sutured to the NG tube. This is withdrawn back into the stomach and the omental plug is then sewn to the edges of the ulcer. In a single randomized trial comparing omental plug with standard omental patch, plug repair was associated with a lower recurrent leak and duodenal stenosis rate.[55] The choice of repair should be influenced by the patient's clinical status, the size of the perforation, the degree of intraperitoneal contamination, and the surgeon's experience.

SUMMARY

Our current understanding of peptic ulcer disease as an infectious disease caused by *H pylori* infection, or a side effect of NSAID use has almost eliminated elective surgery for peptic ulcer disease. However, complications of peptic ulcer disease, either bleeding or perforation, still frequently require surgical intervention. Although bleeding peptic ulcers can usually be treated with nonsurgical means, 5% to 10% will require emergent surgery for hemostasis. With effective medical therapy for peptic ulcer disease, surgical therapy is now focused on obtaining hemostasis and not the underlying ulcer diathesis. Almost all perforated peptic ulcers will require surgery, but the focus of surgery has changed to a damage-control approach rather than one directed at definitive surgical therapy. Although the surgeon does not have to master acid-reducing surgery any longer, emergency ulcer surgery remains high-risk surgery and surgeons must be familiar with the many options for managing this challenging problem.

REFERENCES

1. Paimela H, Paimela L, Myllykangas-Luosujarvi R, et al. Current features of peptic ulcer disease in Finland: incidence of surgery, hospital admissions and mortality for the disease during the past twenty-five years. Scand J Gastroenterol 2002; 37(4):399–403.
2. Schwesinger WH, Page CP, Sirinek KR, et al. Operations for peptic ulcer disease: paradigm lost. J Gastrointest Surg 2001;5(4):438–43.
3. Wang YR, Richter JE, Dempsey DT. Trends and outcomes of hospitalizations for peptic ulcer disease in the United States, 1993 to 2006. Ann Surg 2010;251(1): 51–8.
4. Sarosi GA Jr, Jaiswal KR, Nwariaku FE, et al. Surgical therapy of peptic ulcers in the 21st century: more common than you think. Am J Surg 2005;190(5):775–9.
5. Malfertheiner P, Chan FK, McColl KE. Peptic ulcer disease. Lancet 2009; 374(9699):1449–61.
6. Marshall BJ, Warren JR. Unidentified curved bacilli in the stomach of patients with gastritis and peptic ulceration. Lancet 1984;1(8390):1311–5.
7. NIH Consensus Conference. *Helicobacter pylori* in peptic ulcer disease. NIH Consensus Development Panel on *Helicobacter pylori* in peptic ulcer disease. JAMA 1994;272(1):65–9.
8. Wallace JL. Prostaglandins, NSAIDs, and gastric mucosal protection: why doesn't the stomach digest itself? Physiol Rev 2008;88(4):1547–65.
9. Huang JQ, Sridhar S, Hunt RH. Role of *Helicobacter pylori* infection and non-steroidal anti-inflammatory drugs in peptic-ulcer disease: a meta-analysis. Lancet 2002;359(9300):14–22.
10. Ahsberg K, Ye W, Lu Y, et al. Hospitalisation of and mortality from bleeding peptic ulcer in Sweden: a nationwide time-trend analysis. Aliment Pharmacol Ther 2011; 33(5):578–84.

11. Groenen MJ, Kuipers EJ, Hansen BE, et al. Incidence of duodenal ulcers and gastric ulcers in a Western population: back to where it started. Can J Gastroenterol 2009;23(9):604–8.
12. Barkun AN, Bardou M, Kuipers EJ, et al. International consensus recommendations on the management of patients with nonvariceal upper gastrointestinal bleeding. Ann Intern Med 2010;152(2):101–13.
13. Blatchford O, Murray WR, Blatchford M. A risk score to predict need for treatment for upper-gastrointestinal haemorrhage. Lancet 2000;356(9238):1318–21.
14. Loperfido S, Baldo V, Piovesana E, et al. Changing trends in acute upper-GI bleeding: a population-based study. Gastrointest Endosc 2009;70(2):212–24.
15. Cook DJ, Guyatt GH, Salena BJ, et al. Endoscopic therapy for acute nonvariceal upper gastrointestinal hemorrhage: a meta-analysis. Gastroenterology 1992;102(1):139–48.
16. Sacks HS, Chalmers TC, Blum AL, et al. Endoscopic hemostasis. An effective therapy for bleeding peptic ulcers. JAMA 1990;264(4):494–9.
17. Laine L, McQuaid KR. Endoscopic therapy for bleeding ulcers: an evidence-based approach based on meta-analyses of randomized controlled trials. Clin Gastroenterol Hepatol 2009;7(1):33–47 [quiz: 31–2].
18. Rockall TA, Logan RF, Devlin HB, et al. Risk assessment after acute upper gastro-intestinal haemorrhage. Gut 1996;38(3):316–21.
19. Elmunzer BJ, Young SD, Inadomi JM, et al. Systematic review of the predictors of recurrent hemorrhage after endoscopic hemostatic therapy for bleeding peptic ulcers. Am J Gastroenterol 2008;103(10):2625–32 [quiz: 2633].
20. Morris DL, Hawker PC, Brearley S, et al. Optimal timing of operation for bleeding peptic ulcer: prospective randomised trial. Br Med J (Clin Res Ed) 1984;288(6426):1277–80.
21. Saperas E, Pique JM, Perez Ayuso R, et al. Conservative management of bleeding duodenal ulcer without a visible vessel: prospective randomized trial. Br J Surg 1987;74(9):784–6.
22. Imhof M, Ohmann C, Roher HD, et al. Endoscopic versus operative treatment in high-risk ulcer bleeding patients—results of a randomised study. Langenbecks Arch Surg 2003;387(9–10):327–36.
23. Lau JY, Sung JJ, Lam YH, et al. Endoscopic retreatment compared with surgery in patients with recurrent bleeding after initial endoscopic control of bleeding ulcers. N Engl J Med 1999;340(10):751–6.
24. Hopper AN, Stephens MR, Lewis WG, et al. Relative value of repeat gastric ulcer surveillance gastroscopy in diagnosing gastric cancer. Gastric Cancer 2006;9(3):217–22.
25. Csendes A, Braghetto I, Calvo F, et al. Surgical treatment of high gastric ulcer. Am J Surg 1985;149(6):765–70.
26. Ng EK, Lam YH, Sung JJ, et al. Eradication of *Helicobacter pylori* prevents recurrence of ulcer after simple closure of duodenal ulcer perforation: randomized controlled trial. Ann Surg 2000;231(2):153–8.
27. Gilliam AD, Speake WJ, Lobo DN, et al. Current practice of emergency vagotomy and *Helicobacter pylori* eradication for complicated peptic ulcer in the United Kingdom. Br J Surg 2003;90(1):88–90.
28. Millat B, Hay JM, Valleur P, et al. Emergency surgical treatment for bleeding duodenal ulcer: oversewing plus vagotomy versus gastric resection, a controlled randomized trial. French Associations for Surgical Research. World J Surg 1993;17(5):568–73 [discussion: 574].

29. Poxon VA, Keighley MR, Dykes PW, et al. Comparison of minimal and conventional surgery in patients with bleeding peptic ulcer: a multicentre trial. Br J Surg 1991;78(11):1344–5.
30. Eriksson LG, Ljungdahl M, Sundbom M, et al. Transcatheter arterial embolization versus surgery in the treatment of upper gastrointestinal bleeding after therapeutic endoscopy failure. J Vasc Interv Radiol 2008;19(10):1413–8.
31. Holme JB, Nielsen DT, Funch-Jensen P, et al. Transcatheter arterial embolization in patients with bleeding duodenal ulcer: an alternative to surgery. Acta Radiol 2006;47(3):244–7.
32. Bertleff MJ, Lange JF. Laparoscopic correction of perforated peptic ulcer: first choice? A review of literature. Surg Endosc 2010;24(6):1231–9.
33. Lanas A, Serrano P, Bajador E, et al. Evidence of aspirin use in both upper and lower gastrointestinal perforation. Gastroenterology 1997;112(3):683–9.
34. Gabriel SE, Jaakkimainen L, Bombardier C. Risk for serious gastrointestinal complications related to use of nonsteroidal anti-inflammatory drugs. A meta-analysis. Ann Intern Med 1991;115(10):787–96.
35. Lanza FL. A guideline for the treatment and prevention of NSAID-induced ulcers. Members of the Ad Hoc Committee on Practice Parameters of the American College of Gastroenterology. Am J Gastroenterol 1998;93(11):2037–46.
36. Mort JR, Aparasu RR, Baer RK. Interaction between selective serotonin reuptake inhibitors and nonsteroidal antiinflammatory drugs: review of the literature. Pharmacotherapy 2006;26(9):1307–13.
37. Graham DY, Malaty HM. Alendronate and naproxen are synergistic for development of gastric ulcers. Arch Intern Med 2001;161(1):107–10.
38. Silen W. Cope's early diagnosis of the acute abdomen. 19th edition. New York: Oxford University Press; 1996.
39. Svanes C, Lie RT, Svanes K, et al. Adverse effects of delayed treatment for perforated peptic ulcer. Ann Surg 1994;220(2):168–75.
40. Boey J, Wong J, Ong GB. A prospective study of operative risk factors in perforated duodenal ulcers. Ann Surg 1982;195(3):265–9.
41. Grassi R, Romano S, Pinto A, et al. Gastro-duodenal perforations: conventional plain film, US and CT findings in 166 consecutive patients. Eur J Radiol 2004;50(1):30–6.
42. Lew E. Peptic ulcer disease. In: Greenberger NJ, Blumberg RS, Burakoff R, editors. Current diagnosis & treatment: gastroenterology, hepatology, endoscopy. 1st edition. Columbus (OH): McGraw-Hill; 2009. p. 175–83.
43. Gisbert JP, de la Morena F, Abraira V. Accuracy of monoclonal stool antigen test for the diagnosis of *H. pylori* infection: a systematic review and meta-analysis. Am J Gastroenterol 2006;101(8):1921–30.
44. Leodolter A, Wolle K, Peitz U, et al. Evaluation of a near-patient fecal antigen test for the assessment of *Helicobacter pylori* status. Diagn Microbiol Infect Dis 2004;48(2):145–7.
45. Lee SC, Fung CP, Chen HY, et al. Candida peritonitis due to peptic ulcer perforation: incidence rate, risk factors, prognosis and susceptibility to fluconazole and amphotericin B. Diagn Microbiol Infect Dis 2002;44(1):23–7.
46. Shan YS, Hsu HP, Hsieh YH, et al. Significance of intraoperative peritoneal culture of fungus in perforated peptic ulcer. Br J Surg 2003;90(10):1215–9.
47. Donovan AJ, Berne TV, Donovan JA. Perforated duodenal ulcer: an alternative therapeutic plan. Arch Surg 1998;133(11):1166–71.
48. Crofts TJ, Park KG, Steele RJ, et al. A randomized trial of nonoperative treatment for perforated peptic ulcer. N Engl J Med 1989;320(15):970–3.

49. Moller MH, Shah K, Bendix J, et al. Risk factors in patients surgically treated for peptic ulcer perforation. Scand J Gastroenterol 2009;44(2):145–52, 142 p following 152.
50. Cellan-Jones CJ. A rapid method of treatment in perforated duodenal ulcer. Br Med J 1929;1(3571):1076–7.
51. Siu WT, Leong HT, Law BK, et al. Laparoscopic repair for perforated peptic ulcer: a randomized controlled trial. Ann Surg 2002;235(3):313–9.
52. Johnson AG. Proximal gastric vagotomy: does it have a place in the future management of peptic ulcer? World J Surg 2000;24(3):259–63.
53. Lehnert T, Buhl K, Dueck M, et al. Two-stage radical gastrectomy for perforated gastric cancer. Eur J Surg Oncol 2000;26(8):780–4.
54. McGee GS, Sawyers JL. Perforated gastric ulcers. A plea for management by primary gastric resection. Arch Surg 1987;122(5):555–61.
55. Jani K, Saxena AK, Vaghasia R. Omental plugging for large-sized duodenal peptic perforations: a prospective randomized study of 100 patients. South Med J 2006;99(5):467–71.
56. Lal P, Vindal A, Hadke NS. Controlled tube duodenostomy in the management of giant duodenal ulcer perforation: a new technique for a surgically challenging condition. Am J Surg 2009;198(3):319–23.
57. Gupta S, Kaushik R, Sharma R, et al. The management of large perforations of duodenal ulcers. BMC Surg 2005;5:15.

Gastroesophageal Reflux Disease

Alexander S. Rosemurgy, MD[a,*], Natalie Donn, BS[b,c], Harold Paul, BS[b,c], Kenneth Luberice, BS[b,c], Sharona B. Ross, MD[b,c]

KEYWORDS

• GERD • Gastroesophageal reflux disease
• Laparoendoscopic single-site (LESS) surgery • Fundoplication
• Acid reflux • pH study

Gastroesophageal reflux disease (GERD) has been a significant problem in the United States and around the world for years.[1] Millions of Americans are affected by gastroesophageal reflux in many different ways. Virtually everyone has at least occasional gastroesophageal reflux. However, for millions of Americans gastroesophageal reflux is a significant problem. For them, gastroesophageal reflux imparts tremendous morbidity and at significant cost, not only to their personal health care cost but also to the health care costs of the United States. Given the direct cost of health care delivery to patients with reflux, including medication costs, certainly billions of dollars are spent on the care of GERD annually. When the morbidity and impact of GERD are considered, costs are exponentially higher. When determining the latter costs, time off work, changes in lifestyle, changes in eating and sleeping habits, and impairment of quality of life must be considered.

The magnitude of the problem of GERD was brought to light by the introduction of minimally invasive surgery and the advent of the many medications that are effective in acid suppression. In the 1970s, H_2 blockers began to appear in the armamentarium of physicians. They were liberally prescribed often without objective indications. Liberal application of acid suppressive pharmacotherapy continues. Despite widespread availability of endoscopy and ambulatory pH testing, acid suppressive therapy is generally applied without objective indications. Furthermore, the advent of minimally invasive surgery and, therefore, a less invasive definitive therapy for reflux, has brought another level of consciousness to GERD in the United States. Minimally invasive surgery has resulted in millions of antireflux operations being undertaken, a dramatic, even explosive, increase in the application of surgery for GERD.

The authors have nothing to disclose.

[a] Tampa General Hospital Medical Group, 409 Bayshore Boulevard, Tampa, FL 33606, USA
[b] The Center for Surgical Digestive Disorders, Tampa General Hospital, 2 Columbia Drive, Tampa, FL 33606, USA
[c] Division of General Surgery, College of Medicine, University of South Florida, PO Box 1289, Suite F-145, Tampa, FL 33606, USA
* Corresponding author.
E-mail address: arosemurgy@tgh.org

Surg Clin N Am 91 (2011) 1015–1029
doi:10.1016/j.suc.2011.06.004
surgical.theclinics.com
0039-6109/11/$ – see front matter © 2011 Elsevier Inc. All rights reserved.

The consequences of GERD cannot be denied. Symptoms of reflux, for example heartburn, can be disabling. Many Americans bothered by reflux change their eating and sleeping habits. Patients with GERD may have voice changes associated with reflux. Hoarseness is common. Cough can be brought about by reflux. Furthermore, many Americans may be afflicted by recurring pneumonias as a consequence of reflux and aspiration. Many seek emergency health care for chest pain caused by noncardiac angina such as esophageal spasms brought about by reflux.

Consequences of reflux can also be noted in the dramatic increase in cancer of the esophagus, and specifically at the gastroesophageal junction, in the United States.[2] Barrett esophagus is ever more common as a consequence of GERD. Patients with Barrett esophagus seem more resistant to medical therapy.[3] Often patients with cancer have known gastroesophageal reflux and have received therapy for an extended period of time. Prolonged reflux may lead to esophageal injury and over time to Barrett esophagus and then to dysplasia, leading to a sequence of changes that results in cancer of the esophagus. Precancerous changes in the esophagus, such as Barrett esophagus, should always be considered when caring for patients with long-standing reflux.

The proliferation of potent antiacid medications, such as proton pump inhibitors (PPIs), has exploded worldwide. In the 1970s, H_2 blockers replaced conventional antacid therapy. PPIs have longer half-lives and are more effective in preventing acid secretion than H_2 blockers. The use of PPIs costs billions of dollars per year. In 2009, Nexium had sales of $6.3 billion alone.[4] However, their considerable price transcends beyond just dollars and cents. PPIs increase the risk of community-acquired pneumonia and the risk of *Clostridium difficile* in hospitalized patients. Osteoporosis is a well-recognized complication of prolonged PPI therapy. Given that many patients requiring PPI therapy are women beyond menopause in whom osteoporosis is already a problem, PPI therapy can accelerate their osteoporosis. Osteoporosis with PPI therapy is a problem even in men more than 50 years of age. In addition, PPIs do not stop reflux, they are simply antiacid antisecretory medications. Thus, patients on potent PPI therapy still reflux, although it may not be so acidic. Even if the nonacidic fluid is benign, it can still lead to many complications of reflux including, as has already been mentioned, voice changes, cough, and recurring pneumonia. Furthermore, PPI therapy can prevent the action of some common and important drugs such as Plavix. A proform of Plavix is altered by PPI therapy such that the Plavix is not activated and does not become an active drug. Furthermore, by altering gastric pH, PPIs can interfere with absorption of many drugs and nutrients, such as iron. Cancer associated with the PPI therapy is of increasing concern. PPI therapy can dramatically limit the secretion of gastric acid and ongoing reflux is mostly of unconjugated bile acids. These bile acids are known potent carcinogens and can lead to a sequence of events resulting in adenocarcinoma of the gastroesophageal junction, which is now an epidemic in the United States.[2] PPI therapy can be expensive. Such expense is not limited just to the cost of the drugs but also must include frequent doctor visits for evaluation and care, surveillance endoscopy, and other costs associated with the long-term nonoperative care of reflux, including caring for complications of reflux, such as pneumonia. Viewed in this light, the cost of PPI therapy in the United States is measured in tens of billions of dollars.

WHY DO PEOPLE GET GERD?

Although it is apparent that everybody refluxes occasionally, some patients develop GERD, a condition more advanced than gastroesophageal reflux. There are 3 basic reasons why people get GERD.

Poor Clearance

Poor esophageal clearance allows even occasional reflux to become a severe condition. Again, given that everybody refluxes at least occasionally, most people quickly clear reflux material from their esophagus and no harm is done. However, for patients with poor esophageal clearance, even occasional reflux may result in long dwell times, meaning that gastric acid reflux into the esophagus may persist for a considerable period, causing injury to the esophagus.

Poor esophageal clearance is a monumental although generally uncommon cause of GERD. However, there are no good therapeutic options for patients with poor esophageal clearance. The therapeutic options are limited and include limited operative options. For these patients, generally, PPI therapy is a primary option because it is always best to do no harm; for example, do not do something that results in profound dysphagia. The misapplication of antireflux surgery in patients with poor clearance can be devastating. The construction of a potent gastroesophageal valve mechanism in a patient with a poor esophageal clearance results in profound dysphagia.

Although PPIs do not stop reflux, only acid secretion (to varying degrees), they can be a primary therapy for patients with poor esophageal clearance. Poor esophageal clearance must be considered in everybody with GERD before any invasive intervention; esophageal motility must be determined.

There may be many causes of poor clearance, one of which is a primary motility disorder of the esophagus. This disorder may occur for no apparent reason but is particularly common in older patients, particularly after a stroke, or in patients with collagen vascular disorders, such as scleroderma. However, any form of esophageal obstruction can lead to bizarre or altered motility of the esophagus. For example, a large paraesophageal hernia could impair esophageal emptying and, in time, lead to altered esophageal motility. These causes must be considered in patients who have altered motility patterns because relief of obstruction may allow for the return of normal motility, in contrast to patients with achalasia in whom motility disturbance is a sine qua non of the disease.

Poor Gastric Emptying

Poor gastric emptying can cause GERD. If the stomach does not empty as it fills up, ultimately gastric contents spill back into the esophagus. Gastric emptying should be determined in the course of evaluation of patients with GERD. It may not be necessary to undertake a specific test of gastric emptying, like a gastric emptying scan, but poor gastric emptying must be considered when patients have retained gastric contents at the time of endoscopy after a prolonged period of nothing by mouth.

Gastric emptying scans in the evaluation of gastric emptying need to be interpreted with caution. Gastroesophageal reflux caused by a poor lower esophageal sphincter (LES) mechanism can be a cause of prolonged gastric emptying. In patients with severe reflux, gastric pressures are vented up into the esophagus with gastric contents with gastric contractions and increases in intragastric pressures. Emptying backwards into the esophagus may be the path of least resistance, with less resistance than emptying down into the duodenum through the pylorus. Therefore, an antireflux procedure may dramatically improve gastric emptying. It is not gastric emptying that needs to be determined before invasive procedures, but the presence of gastric contractility and antral/pyloric patency. Contrast studies of the upper gastrointestinal (GI) tract, including the esophagus and stomach, and upper endoscopy are helpful in determining anatomic problems that could be confused with primary motility disturbances. Anatomic problems, such as pyloric stenosis, require their specific corrections.

Poor emptying by gastric emptying scan is often reported to be gastroparesis. Gastric emptying scans may show delayed gastric emptying in patients with notable gastroesophageal reflux. An interpretation of gastroparesis must be interpreted with caution. It is our practice to follow an abnormal gastric emptying scan with an upper GI tract contrast study to ascertain gastric contractility and patency of gastric outlet. If the stomach contracts normally with an anatomically normal outlet, and without other concerns such as retained food on gastroscopy, then delayed gastric emptying is attributed to gastroesophageal reflux.

Poor Gastroesophageal Valve (Poor LES)

The foremost cause, and usually the cause considered first, of GERD is a poor valve between the esophagus and the stomach. Although this is the usual cause of gastroesophageal reflux and GERD, it is not the only cause; as mentioned earlier, poor esophageal clearance and poor gastric emptying also need to be considered. Conversely, a poor valve is the most easily corrected cause of GERD and therefore most of the attention in the therapeutic considerations of GERD focuses on the construction of a new or better valve mechanism. This is the premise behind antireflux surgery.

There are not many ways to determine the function or integrity of the LES. Manometry and impedance are not commonly used. However, the LES may be manometrically normal and yet not function well because of transient relaxation. A manometrically normal LES should not deter the application of necessary antireflux surgery.[5]

DIAGNOSIS OF GERD

Symptoms of GERD

The symptoms of GERD are many and can be divided into 2 basic groups: esophageal and extraesophageal symptoms. Esophageal symptoms or manifestations of GERD generally focus on heartburn. Heartburn can occur many times per day. Heartburn may be postprandial or nocturnal. Patients who experience heartburn as a primary symptom generally do best with therapy, medical or operative. Patients with nonesophageal symptoms of reflux often have problems that are the most difficult to treat and ameliorate, particularly because the symptoms may not be acid related but may be related to reflux of even nonacidic material.

Nonesophageal symptoms of reflux can be varied and include, but are not limited to, chest pain, cough, aspiration, pneumonia, hoarseness, sinus problems, and so on. These symptoms may not necessarily be acid related but may be related to reflux of even benign nonacidic fluid. Chronic aspiration associated with nonacid reflux can lead to recurring pneumonias and ultimately pulmonary deterioration. It is important to determine whether or not symptoms of GERD are acid or nonacid related because nonacid-related symptoms do not improve on PPI therapy. These patients require cessation of reflux. Those patients with the best responses to PPI therapy do best with antireflux surgery because they have shown that relief of acid reflux relieves their symptoms. For them, PPI therapy is a successful therapeutic trial.

Esophagoscopy

Esophagoscopy is a useful measure in the diagnosis of GERD. Early evidence of GERD may be erythema in the esophagus. In patients with more advanced reflux disease, esophagitis, erosive esophagitis, and even ulcerations within the esophagus may be notable findings. For patients with long-standing disease, strictures within the esophagus may be noted, because ulcerations may have led to healing with contracture and narrowing of the esophagus. Stricture formation is a finding of chronic reflux and is a disappointing finding with great implications. Often, stricture formation represents end-stage disease and is associated with profound distortion of esophageal motility, which in turn limits application of minimally invasive definitive therapy. It is important for patients with strictures to undergo early and repeated dilation to relieve the stricture and allow for definitive stretching of the esophagus. This practice requires a program of sequential dilation that continues even after cessation of reflux (eg, after fundoplication) with continued dilation until maturation of the scar occurs in a form that allows the patient to be free from dysphagia.

Upper Gastroesophageal Contrast Studies

There is much to be gained from an upper GI contrast study, particularly one performed with thought and care by an engaged radiologist. Such a study can detail anatomy, give great insight into esophageal motility, detect gastric contractions, define the anatomy of the gastric outlet, and detect clinically occult diseases, such as an ulcer. The importance of an upper GI contrast study cannot be overemphasized and it is an essential component of our diagnostic algorithm. However, some findings require restraint, for example, the finding of a hiatal hernia.

Hiatal hernia is not a sine qua non of gastroesophageal reflux or GERD. Hiatal hernia is a common finding and tens of millions of Americans have hiatal hernias. A hiatal hernia should be considered anatomically normal in patients more than 50 years of age, particularly those who are overweight. GERD occurs in a few patients with a hiatal hernia. Stated differently, a hiatal hernia is not a disease state but rather a condition of normalcy. The term hiatal hernia was introduced into the lexicon of Americans in the 1950s and is often believed to be significant, but it denotes no significance in the absence of excess acid reflux or esophageal emptying limitations.

We find that having a patient swallow a barium-laden food bolus in a 15° Trendelenburg position is helpful in determining esophageal motility and emptying. If the bite-size food bolus clears in 2 or fewer stripping motions, esophageal motility is normal. If not, esophageal motility is impaired. We find this study to be more specific than manometry and it is well tolerated by patients.[6]

Ambulatory pH Study

Ambulatory pH studies are an essential part of the diagnosis with patients with reflux. The criteria of normal, as opposed to abnormal, are clear. A DeMeester score is a commonly used measure of reflux.[7] A score of more than 14.7 denotes excess acid reflux. The DeMeester score is calculated by using a host of measures, in both the upright and supine position, which include the frequency of episodes of reflux, the percentage of time with a pH less than 4 in the distal esophagus, the duration of the longest episode of reflux, and the number of acid reflux episodes lasting more than 5 minutes. A score of 6.9 or less is normal. A gray zone exists between 6.9 and 14.7. A score of more than 14.7 is abnormal. Other measures of excess acid reflux rather than DeMeester scores are used by some. Nonsurgeons are more inclined to use percentage of time with a pH less than 4 in the distal esophagus, which is a component of the DeMeester score.

The length of ambulatory pH study should be as long as possible. There are advantages to a 48-hour study as opposed to a 24-hour study, because many patients with gastroesophageal reflux may have episodic excess reflux and that may not be picked up with a 24-hour study. Current technology limits us to ambulatory studies of 48 hours. Ambulatory pH studies can be undertaken through a transnasal approach or through an approach that uses a chip placed onto the distal esophagus. The latter (ie, Bravo pH study) is our preferred approach because it allows patients to assume a more normal lifestyle during the course of study. However, the chip often is associated with notable dysphagia and can render patients uncomfortable during the time of study. However, it seems unlikely that patients with a chip are more uncomfortable than patients with a catheter emanating from their nose. It is important that ambulatory pH studies be undertaken during optimal (ie, usual life activity) circumstances. The patient should be off antiacid medications (such as PPI therapy) well in advance of their studies and during the course of their studies. Ambulatory pH studies undertaken with patients on medication may be normal. Excess acid reflux is not detected because the reflux is nonacidic given the suppression of acid by the PPIs. There is generally no reason to study patients on PPI therapy or other antiacid antisecretory medications.

Ambulatory pH studies should not be undertaken until patients are ready for intervention. For example, patients who need to lose considerable amounts of weight before intervention should not be studied until after their weight loss. Gastric acid secretion is proportional to body mass. As patients lose weight they secret less acid. Furthermore, gastroesophageal reflux is proportional to intra-abdominal pressures, which are directly transmitted to the lumen of the stomach. Heavy patients have high intragastric pressures that promote gastroesophageal reflux. Excessively heavy patients are not good candidates for antireflux surgery. Therefore, patients should not be studied until they are ready for an operation, for example, until they have lost the necessary amount of weight. Furthermore, ambulatory pH studies should be undertaken under usual life activities. They should not be undertaken in such a way that patients after application of the testing device are sent home to rest and be quiet. Active patients should be active during their period of pH testing so that their usual life activities are reflected in their test results. As a caveat, acid pH testing does not detect nonacid reflux. Patients who have nonacidic reflux and complications of nonacid reflux do not have abnormal ambulatory pH testing.

Esophageal Impedance Testing

Esophageal impedance is a relatively new technique developed to detect intraluminal bolus movement. This technique is based on measuring the resistance to alternating current (ie, impedance) of the content of the esophageal lumen.[8] The impedance stays at its lowest point as long as the food bolus is present in the impedance-measuring segment and returns to its baseline once the bolus is cleared by a contraction. Liquid-containing boluses with an increased number of ions conduct higher electrical currents than gases, because of their poor electrical conductance.

Impedance testing is not able to detect the acid content or volume of the intraluminal contents. When combined with pH testing, the detection of both acid and nonacid is permitted and this method is typically more sensitive than pH monitoring alone. Furthermore, when combined with manometry it provides information about both the pressures and bolus transit within the esophagus. Limitations on impedance monitoring can include low baseline impedance values by the mucosa of Barrett esophagus and esophagitis, which make detection of reflux inaccurate in such circumstances. These inaccuracies require manual data correction when using the current automated analysis software.

Impedance testing is most useful in detecting nonacid reflux[9] and is used to detect reflux in patients not responding to PPI therapy or those with normal ambulatory 24-hour or 48-hour pH testing. Impedance testing is also helpful in detecting postprandial reflux, when gastric contents are nonacidic.[9] Impedance testing may provide a superior link between reflux and symptoms than ambulatory pH testing, especially in children.

Manometry

Manometry is generally not an effective tool for a diagnosis of gastroesophageal reflux. Although manometry determines motility patterns that are important in the application of definitive therapy for reflux, reflux and motility patterns of the esophagus may be completely unrelated and unassociated. Therefore, manometry has a role in determining applications of therapy but not in diagnosis of reflux.

INDICATIONS FOR APPLICATION OF DEFINITIVE THERAPY

Symptoms

Control of symptoms is a primary indication for intervention in patients with GERD. The symptoms that indicate intervention must be reflux related. As noted earlier, these symptoms can be divided into 2 groups: esophageal and extraesophageal symptoms of reflux. The differentiation between esophageal and extraesophageal symptoms is an important consideration because they may have different responses to treatment.

Esophageal symptoms of reflux generally mean heartburn. Heartburn is generally relieved with cessation of reflux and acid reflux in particular.

Extraesophageal manifestations of reflux are many and varied. Extraesophageal symptoms include cough, reflux-induced asthma, pulmonary symptoms of aspiration including recurring pneumonia, reflux-induced sinus problems, chest pain, and hoarseness. Relative to heartburn, extraesophageal manifestations of reflux are not so well treated by cessation of acid reflux.[10,11]

PPI therapy is effective in treating esophageal manifestations of reflux, for example, heartburn. Patients who do best with antireflux surgery are patients who do well with PPI therapy because the cessation of symptoms on medical therapy implies or denotes that sensation of reflux through intervention ameliorates symptoms. Patients with hoarseness and cough have a lower response to therapy than do patients with heartburn.[10,11] Nearly 100% of patients with heartburn who respond to PPI therapy have complete relief of symptoms with antireflux surgery. For example, the relief seen in cough is less frequent probably because there are many causes of cough. Only about 70% of patients with excess acid reflux and cough see an improvement in their cough or relief of their cough with relief of the acid reflux through antireflux surgery despite a thorough workup of cough before antireflux surgery. Cough is a symptom that may have many causes, reflux being one, and patients with reflux may also have concomitant allergies or other problems that manifest as cough. Relief of the acid reflux may not provide significant amelioration of cough or other extraesophageal manifestations of reflux despite thorough preoperative evaluation. This observation must be considered in the informed consent process.

Endoscopic Indications

There are endoscopic indications for intervention for reflux. Patients may be asymptomatic and in the surveillance endoscopy they are found to have esophagitis and other findings caused by acid reflux. Patients may not have symptoms because their esophagus is insensate to acid reflux. Patients may not have symptoms but may be noted to have other issues that lead to endoscopy, such as occult GI bleeding. As mentioned earlier, the finding of Barrett esophagus on endoscopy is a more ominous finding than esophagitis.

Esophagitis is a spectrum. It can be found in several different stages, from simple erythema to erosions progressing onto ulcers. Esophagitis is an acute event, in general. The finding of Barrett esophagus denotes long-standing severe reflux. In patients with less than high-grade dysplasia, Barrett esophagus is generally treated with antireflux measures, including fundoplication. However, patients with high-grade dysplasia warrant further intervention beyond the cessation of reflux. The risk of cancer in patients with high-grade dysplasia is such that ablation of the Barrett esophagus or other interventions are necessary. These interventions can include mucosal ablation, endoscopic mucosal resection, or even, in some patients, esophagectomy.

Complaints of dysphagia or the identification of a stricture on endoscopy in a patient with reflux are particularly ominous. Any patients complaining of dysphagia in the presence of reflux have to be considered to have cancer until proved otherwise. The finding of the stricture denotes long-standing severe reflux. The strictures have to be dilatable for antireflux measures alone to be considered. For patients with non-dilatable strictures, esophagectomy is necessary. For a stricture to occur in a patient while on medical therapy is unacceptable, and the practitioner should be accountable for the progression of reflux, and the development of such a severe complication while the patient is under their observation. This situation can be a criticism of medical therapy.

In considering antireflux surgery, the stricture should be dilatable; dilation should be frequent and sufficient to allow for dilation to a significant size, for example, a 56-French to 60-French bougie. In patients undergoing definitive antireflux therapy, such as a fundoplication, a plan for dilation after fundoplication must be formulated preoperatively such that dilations after fundoplication are initially undertaken frequently albeit at an ever-decreasing frequency. This process is so that maturation of the scar can occur with a lumen of adequate size. Even although the reflux has been relieved after fundoplication, the healing process continues, reflecting prefundoplication reflux. Dilation, given the severity of the stricture, may need to continue for up to several years after eradication of the reflux, albeit in an ever-decreasing frequency.

Persistent Symptoms Despite Medications

Patients may have symptoms caused by reflux despite antireflux medications such as PPIs. For these patients, definitive resolution of their reflux is important and they require more than antiacid therapy. These patients need antireflux therapy, not antiacid therapy. For patients who have nonesophageal symptoms of reflux their symptoms are often related to nonacid reflux, and therefore cessation of reflux, not just cessation of acid reflux, is important. These patients require more than just PPI therapy. Their options include endoscopic or laparoscopic fundoplication.

Strictures

Patients with esophageal strictures have developed a severe complication of acid reflux and we believe they should undergo repeated dilation with definitive resolution of gastroesophageal reflux. Although patients generally may do well on PPI therapy, acid suppression is not 24 hours per day. Patients may have therapy twice per day with PPIs, but then costs become considerable and other complications such as osteoporosis become paramount; we believe that patients noted to have strictures caused by reflux are best served by definitive antireflux intervention and therapy directed at their stricture, namely dilation. This dilation needs to continue postoperatively to arrest the structuring process that began preoperatively.

Bleeding Caused by Reflux

Patients noted to have bleeding should undergo endoscopy for documentation of the cause and the bleeding site, and initiation of PPI therapy. Once patients are stable and the bleeding is completely under control, the decision for PPI therapy, as opposed to definitive therapy, needs to be undertaken. Patients with a life-threatening or significant complication associated with reflux require open-ended long-standing therapy and are exposed to all the consequences associated with prolonged PPI therapy, and therefore are best considered as candidates for definitive antireflux therapy.

Barrett Esophagus

Patients with Barrett esophagus are best treated with definitive antireflux therapy. PPI therapy is not uniformly efficacious in acid suppression and these patients require open-ended therapy. Given that there is a path along which esophageal injury occurs, Barrett esophagus represents a relatively advanced manifestation of reflux, and patients are best served by having definitive antireflux intervention. After cessation of acid reflux, regression of Barrett esophagus is possible.[12]

Cost of Care

The costs of medication, follow-up, medical care, and endoscopy have to be considered in the decision to intervene and provide definitive antireflux therapy. For patients with projected open-ended therapy, the cost, inconvenience, risk of complications, and compliance necessary for long-term care and follow-up are considerable, and definitive antireflux therapy should be given early consideration. If there is a medically treatable cause of reflux or a treatable factor that exacerbates reflux, such as obesity, then PPI therapy seems indicated even in young patients until the treatable causes can be brought under control or treated. However, for young, thin, healthy patients without notable risk factors for GERD, antireflux surgery should be an early consideration.

Compliance

Definitive antireflux therapy, and specifically antireflux surgery, should be considered for patients who are unavailable or do not cooperate with ongoing medical care and follow-up.

General Conditions

Patients who do best with definitive acid reflux therapy (ie, laparoscopic fundoplication) are patients who do best with PPI therapy. It is also important to consider that before intervention numerous steps should be undertaken.

Before intervention is undertaken, medical therapy should be undertaken while treatments of comorbidities are evaluated. As stated earlier, a PPI therapy is a great predictor of patients who do well with definitive antireflux intervention. PPI therapy is, in a sense, a therapeutic trial, particularity given heartburn and other esophageal symptoms of GERD.

If it is possible to ameliorate causative factors associated with reflux before intervention, it should be undertaken. For example, patients who are heavy should lose weight. We look for a body mass index (BMI, calculated as weight in kilograms divided by the square of height in meters) of less than 26 kg/m^2 before any definitive intervention is considered. Weight loss decreases acid secretion, and as mentioned earlier, it decreases intragastric pressures, which leads to less of a driving force for acid gastroesophageal reflux.

Patients who smoke should stop. They should change this lifestyle that promotes gastroesophageal reflux. For example, a lifestyle that involves inducing high intragastric pressures should change. Patients should avoid methylated xanthenes (eg, chocolate) and alcohol. Furthermore, they should not function at high altitudes or lower atmospheric pressures, if possible. It is simplistic to say that these measures should be undertaken, but some patients find it impossible; someone cannot move from Denver, Colorado to a city at sea level just to avoid reflux. Intervention may be necessary because of a life at higher altitudes. However, if reflux occurs in a patient who only intermittently travels to higher altitudes, where reflux can be excessive,[13] several weeks of PPI therapy per year are a small price to pay to control intermittent reflux.

Once someone has been optimized for intervention, then appropriate evaluation of their reflux should be undertaken. Ambulatory pH studies should not be undertaken while patients are heavy but rather after they have lost the appropriate weight. Esophageal motility needs to be determined.

Patients and their care providers should understand the disease process for each patient. Upper GI contrast studies for determination of causes of symptoms are important. Upper endoscopy should also be undertaken before intervention to rule out other diseases and to evaluate for Barrett esophagus, and to determine gastric emptying (ie, residual food) and gastric outlet. The upper GI study mentioned earlier should be used to look for gastric contractions and gastric emptying. Gastric emptying scans are not necessary in most patients and are often overinterpreted. Delayed gastric emptying in a patient with reflux may simply be caused by excess gastroesophageal reflux. Nonetheless, nuclear medicine physicians generally report delayed gastric emptying as equating to gastroparesis, further complicating the patient's care. Delayed gastric emptying may not be related to gastroparesis at all. The delayed gastric emptying may be nothing more than a manifestation of notable gastroesophageal reflux.

It is important to understand esophageal motility before intervention. Esophageal motility can be determined through manometry, impedance, or, as in our choice, a barium-laden food bolus with the patient in a 15° head-down position. This position allows us to determine anatomy, esophageal motility, and gastric contractility and emptying. This study requires that a food bolus, like a bite of a marshmallow or bagel, be cleared from the esophagus by 1 to 2 stripping motions. If a barium-laden food bolus is cleared with 2 or fewer stripping motions, patients do well after fundoplication, with a low incidence of dysphagia.[6] We find that this is a better measure of esophageal function than manometry, which seems too sensitive.[6]

Impedance testing, and high-definition impedance testing in particular, is the newest testing modality to be widely studied. Early studies with impedance testing are promising and seem to be sensitive and specific when determining esophageal motility. Such testing can detect nonacidic bolus reflux.

A full evaluation of all comorbidities must be undertaken before any intervention is considered or initiated. Risks of the intervention must be estimated and efforts must be undertaken to decrease risk. For example, for a patient with inducible cardiac ischemia, revascularization with either stenting or bypassing must be undertaken before intervention for reflux disease. In general, medical comorbidities and age should not deter the application of laparoscopic fundoplication.[14,15]

Informed Consent

The informed consent process should be detailed and specific, as before any operation or any intervention. There are 8 complaints that commonly occur after antireflux surgery and we are specific about telling patients about these, which we learned from the more than 1000 patients on whom we have performed fundoplications. These 8 complaints are:

1. Shoulder pain, probably caused by pneumoperitoneum.
2. Dysphagia caused by swelling at the gastroesophageal junction associated with the dissection and construction of the valve mechanism.
3. Bloating associated with aerophagia. Aerophagia is associated with dry swallowing, which patients do excessively preoperatively to induce esophageal motility

to clear their refluxed material. This is a learned behavior and patients continue to do it after the operation; they swallow a lot of air (ie, aerophagia), which leads to notable bloating and other symptoms. This behavior is unlearned in time. To lessen bloating, patients should not chew gum or drink with straws.

4. Flatulence. This is a consequence as well of aerophagia because patients do not belch or reflux so much after fundoplication. Bloating and flatulence are a consequence of aerophagia and the iatrogenic limitation of belching.
5. Diarrhea. This condition is really better stated as defecatory frequency; whatever it is called, it is a consequence of the aerophagia, bloating, and air in the intestinal tract. As intestinal motility picks up to more rapidly clear the air descending in the bowel, increased flatulence is a consequence, as is defecatory frequency. Attempts to control defecatory frequency with medications such as Imodium increase bloating. Patients cannot be counseled on decreasing aerophagia, it decreases with time. Aerophagia is a subconsciously learned behavior and is unlearned with time.
6. Nausea. Again, this is probably a consequence of aerophagia.
7. Early satiety. Early satiety is a consequence of a smaller gastric reservoir, which is a result of the stomach being used in the antireflux procedure, and is a consequence of notable aerophagia, which may leave the patient with a stomach full of air when the first bite of food is taken.
8. Incisional pain. This complaint is aided by injecting local anesthesia into the umbilicus before the incision is made.

Informed consent must also consider that there are failures in control of symptoms associated with reflux, which is particularly true with patients who have nonesophageal symptoms of reflux. There may also be some new symptoms after fundoplication, such as dysphagia.

INTERVENTION BEYOND MEDICAL THERAPY

Interventions beyond medical therapy can generally be divided into 2 basic groups: endoscopic and laparoscopic. The days of open procedures need to be considered as a thing of the past. However, the possibility of open surgery should be noted in the consent.

Endoscopic

Endoscopic therapy generally is limited to EsophyX (EndoGastric Solutions, Inc, Redmond, WA), often called transoral incisionless fundoplication. EsophyX is a transoral approach to an endoscopic placation of the esophagogastric junction to construct a more prominent gastroesophageal flap valve, much in the manner of an endoscopic Belsey Mark IV procedure. Using EsophyX, a rotational longitudinal esophagogastric fundoplication is constructed.[16] Using EsophyX, a full-thickness esophagogastric fundoplication is constructed with fixation extending longitudinally 3.5 cm above the Z-line and rotationally more than 270° around the esophagus.

Although it has been studied in many different ways manometrically and is often compared with a Nissen fundoplication, EsophyX seems to be more of an endoscopic approach to the Belsey Mark IV procedure. It does not really limit esophageal emptying or act to impede esophageal emptying and in patients with esophageal dysmotility it probably serves as a preferred alternative to other procedures, given documented efficacy, such as Nissen fundoplication. Candidates for EsophyX should be in good health and of ideal body size (eg, BMI <30 kg/m^2), as mentioned earlier, and have a hiatal hernia less than 2 cm in size.

Although it is heavily marketed, there are not many data regarding long-term outcomes associated with EsophyX. There are few controlled data. Patients who have undergone EsophyX therapy generally have a reduced use of PPI therapy. Many have control of their acid reflux, although generally only a few. Early results show that 37% to 49% of patients have normalization of acid exposure to the esophagus.[17] Resting pressures of the LES are also improved.[17]

An increasing number of patients are being treated, and results of long-term outcomes are still being determined. Revisions after EsophyX are not problematic, and favorable outcomes can be expected after revisional laparoscopic fundoplications.[18]

Controlled trials of EsophyX would be helpful in determining its place in the armamentarium of antireflux surgery.

Laparoscopic Fundoplication

The gold standard for intervention is laparoscopic fundoplication. What type of laparoscopic fundoplication is chosen is at the discretion of the surgeon. Debate continues as to which is the best type of fundoplication, with many differing opinions.[19] We believe, as do others, that fundoplication controls acid reflux better than PPIs.[20–24] Generally, normal esophageal motility dictates that a Nissen fundoplication be undertaken and a Toupet fundoplication be undertaken for patients with altered or minimally to moderately impaired esophageal motility. Patients with no esophageal motility would probably do poorly with whatever fundoplication were chosen and are best not operated on. Again, first do no harm. An example of a patient in this category is a patient with scleroderma or a collagen vascular disorder severely limiting esophageal motility. Those patients are best served by avoiding fundoplication in its entirety and continuing to receive therapy with a PPI, if possible. Although PPI therapy may not be perfect or ideal for those patients, dysphagia is a morbid symptom, and patients are unhappy if dysphagia is augmented or induced by fundoplication.

Before undertaking laparoscopic fundoplication, remember that the best candidates for laparoscopic fundoplication are those who are in good health and those who did well with PPI therapy.

The goals of laparoscopic fundoplication are (1) to reduce the hiatal hernia in its entirety, (2) to mobilize 8 cm of esophagus into the abdomen, and (3) to construct a valve mechanism. Furthermore, the gastric outlet needs to be ensured. This objective is best achieved preoperatively by endoscopy or barium study.

Our technique of fundoplication involves several basic steps. The gastrohepatic omentum is opened in a stellate fashion to allow wide visualization of the right crus and to facilitate rolling of the stomach from left to right. The dissection should be carried up and down the right crus, then into the mediastinum, and any hiatal hernia should begin to be reduced. The stomach should then be rolled to the right and the short gastric vessels divided. The dissection should be carried to the left crus, up and down the crus, and then into the mediastinum. The hiatal hernia should be reduced in its entirety and the hiatal hernia sac excised as much as possible, with care not to injure the vagal fibers. The gastroesophageal fat pad should be excised. The esophageal hiatus should be reconstructed with a posterior cruroplasty so that it is snug, but not tight, about the esophagus. Mesh may be necessary to provide for a secure reconstruction of the hiatus. It is not in our routine to use mesh. If mesh is used it should be a bioprosthesis and not polypropylene mesh. We use the bioprosthesis to reinforce an insecure closure or to augment a closure that is not otherwise possible when the left and right crura cannot be opposed. The latter occurrence is very uncommon and the former is relatively uncommon. Some use a bioprosthesis for reconstruction of the hiatus with patients with paraesophageal hernias and some use it routinely. There are data to support this approach,[25] but the expense of mesh, complications associated with mesh (ie, infection, dysphagia), and the success of our approach have caused us to use mesh infrequently.

Once the hiatus has been reconstructed, a valve mechanism is constructed. Generally we construct a Nissen fundoplication in patients with normal esophageal motility. We construct a Nissen fundoplication, securing the anterior fundus and the posterior fundus to the esophagus twice, with the sutures placed well above the gastroesophageal junction. A third suture approximates the anterior fundus and the posterior fundus at the level of the gastroesophageal junction. This fundoplication is undertaken with a bougie through the mouth in the stomach: size 52 to 56 French in women and size 56 to 60 French in men. Once the valve is constructed and the bougie removed, the posterior fundus is tacked to the right side of the esophagus and then to the right crus so that there is no tension promoting the wrap to come undone or twisting to the esophagus.

It is now our preferred approach to use a laparoendoscopic single-site (LESS) approach. This approach uses only a 12-mm incision at the umbilicus. This incision provides optimal cosmesis and a speedy return to normal functional activities. To operate on patients and leave no notable scar is, by any measure, outstanding. Our results with laparoscopic fundoplications are consistent with many others.[26–30] Our results with LESS fundoplication are similar to with laparoscopic fundoplication.[31] Our results and the results of many others document the salutary benefits of antireflux surgery and promote further application.

Millions of patients have undergone laparoscopic antireflux surgery. We believe that results recommend continued application. Success is uniform and durable. However, success is not universal. Patients fail. Under the best of circumstances and in the best of surgical practices, patients fail for many reasons. Some of them may be related to patients' behavior, such as coughing or vomiting postoperatively. Some of them may be related to some subtle failure in technique that is not apparent to the operating surgeon. For example, in a given patient the fundoplication may be constructed too tight or with too much tension, leading to postoperative dysphagia. In another patient, a secure hiatal reconstruction may fail. Failure may occur for no apparent reason, but on long-term follow-up, unraveling of the wrap or failure of the hiatal reconstruction may be noted. Failure is uncommon. Postoperative paraesophageal hernias occur infrequently. The same is true for sliding hiatal hernias. It should be noted whether they are important and whether they are true failures as opposed to incidental findings. For example, a 2-cm hiatal hernia after fundoplication may be a finding on an upper GI study that has no notable clinical significance. Many would consider this as a normal finding, given that most people more than 60 years of age have at least a small hiatal hernia.

Patients should be followed up with ambulatory pH testing, which should be used as a gold standard for reflux.[32] Patients should be followed up with an upper GI study to be used as a measure of anatomic normalcy. However, ambulatory pH studies are the true measure of acid reflux and findings of upper GI studies must not be considered significant for reflux; anatomic findings on an upper GI study cannot be subtle and important. To be important, findings must be truly notable and noteworthy. An example of a noteworthy finding is a large paraesophageal hernia or a large hiatal hernia, which may lead to other symptoms. A 2-cm hiatal hernia could be an anatomic normalcy and denotes no significance in a postoperative period. Symptomatic control of patients with reflux has proved to be durable and satisfactory.

Control of acid reflux by ambulatory pH testing after fundoplication is noted to be satisfactory and durable, although patients are generally unwilling to undergo surveillance pH testing. Laparoscopic fundoplication has established itself as the gold standard for the control of reflux.

Measures beyond fundoplication such as esophagectomy should be considered in patients only with notable complications, such as cancer or nondilatable stricture formation, as noted earlier.

REFERENCES

1. Sontag SJ. The medical management of reflux esophagitis: role of antacids and acid inhibition. Surg Clin North Am 1990;19:683–712.
2. Altekruse SF, Kosary CL, Krapcho M, et al. SEER cancer statistics review, 1975–2007. Bethesda (MD): National Cancer Institute; November 2009. Available at: http://seer.cancer.gov/csr/1975_2007/. Accessed 2010.
3. DeVault KR, Castell DO. Updated guidelines for the diagnosis and treatment of gastroesophageal reflux disease. Am J Gastroenterol 2005;100:190–200.
4. Drugs to treat heartburn and acid reflux: the proton pump inhibitors comparing effectiveness, safety, and pumps. Available at: http://consumerreports.org/health/resources/pdf/best-buy-drugs/PPIsUpdate-FINAL.pdf. Updated May 2010. Accessed February 28, 2011.
5. Cowgill SM, Bloomston M, Al-Saadi S, et al. Normal lower esophageal sphincter pressure and length does not impact outcome after laparoscopic Nissen fundoplication. J Gastrointest Surg 2007;6:701–7.
6. D'Alessio MJ, Rakita S, Bloomston M, et al. Esophagography predicts favorable outcome after Nissen fundoplication for patients with esophageal dysmotility. J Am Coll Surg 2005;201:335–42.
7. Johnson LF, DeMeester TR. Twenty-four hour pH monitoring of the distal esophagus. A quantitative measure of gastroesophageal reflux. Am J Gastroenterol 1974;62:325–32.
8. Radu T, Castell DO. Esophageal multichannel intraluminal impedance testing. Available at: http://www.uptodate.com/contents/esophageal-multichannel-intraluminal-impedance-testing. Updated July 22, 2009. Accessed February 19, 2011.
9. Mousa HM, Rosen R, Woodley FW, et al. Esophageal impedance monitoring for gastroesophageal reflux. J Pediatr Gastroenterol Nutr 2011;52(2):129–39.
10. Rakita S, Villadolid D, Thomas A, et al. Laparoscopic Nissen fundoplication offers high patient satisfaction with relief of extra-esophageal symptoms of GERD. Am Surg 2006;72:207–12.
11. Kirkby-Bott J, Jones E, Perring S, et al. Proximal acid reflux treated by fundoplication predicts a good outcome for chronic cough attributable to gastroesophageal reflux disease. Arch Surg 2011;396:167–71.
12. Rosemurgy AS. What's new in surgery: gastrointestinal conditions. J Am Coll Surg 2003;197:792–801.
13. Kumar S, Sharma S, Norboo T, et al. Population based study to assess prevalence and risk factors of gastroesophageal reflux disease in high altitude area. Indian J Gastroenterol 2011;30(3):135–43.
14. Golkar F, Morton C, Ross S, et al. Medical comorbidities should not deter the application of laparoscopic fundoplication. J Gastrointest Surg 2010;14:1214–9.
15. Cowgill SM, Arnaoutakis D, Villadolid D, et al. Results after laparoscopic fundoplication: does age matter? Am Surg 2006;72:778–83.
16. Bell RC, Cadiere GB. Transoral rotational esophagogastric fundoplication: technical, anatomical, and safety considerations. Surg Endosc 2011;25(7):2387–99.
17. Cadiere GB, Buset M, Muls V, et al. Transoral incisionless fundoplication using EsophyX: 12-month results of a prospective multicenter study. World J Surg 2008;32:1676–88.

18. Romario UF, Barbera R, Repici A, et al. Nissen fundoplication after failure of endoluminal fundoplication: short-term results. J Gastrointest Surg 2011;15:439–43.
19. Lundell L. Surgical therapy of gastroesophageal reflux disease. Best Pract Res Clin Gastroenterol 2010;24:947–59.
20. Lundell L, Myrvold HE, Perderson SA, et al. Continued (5-year) follow up of a randomized clinical study comparing antireflux surgery and omeprazole in gastroesophageal reflux disease. J Am Coll Surg 2001;192:172–9.
21. Lundell L, Miettinen P, Myrwold ME, et al. Medical or surgical treatment of reflux esophagitis: 7 year follow up of a randomized clinical trial. Br J Surg 2007;94: 198–203.
22. Lundell L, Miettinen P, Myrwold ME, et al. Comparison of outcomes twelve years after antireflux surgery or omeprazole maintenance therapy for reflux esophagitis. Clin Gastroenterol Hepatol 2009;7:1292–8.
23. Grant AM, Wileman SM, Ramsay CR, et al. Minimal access surgery compared with medical management for chronic gastro-esophageal reflux disease: UK collaborative randomized trail. BMJ 2008;337:a2664.
24. Mehta S, Bennet J, Mahon D, et al. Prospective trial of laparoscopic Nissen fundoplication versus proton pump inhibitor therapy for gastroesophageal reflux disease: seven-year follow-up. J Gastrointest Surg 2006;10:1312–7.
25. Granderath FA, Schweiger UM, Kamolz T, et al. Laparoscopic Nissen fundoplication with prosthetic hiatal closure reduces postoperative intrathoracic wrap herniation: preliminary results of a prospective randomized functional and clinical study. Arch Surg 2005;140:40–8.
26. Bloomston M, Nields W, Rosemurgy AS. Symptoms and antireflux medication use following laparoscopic Nissen fundoplication: outcome at 1 and 4 years. JSLS 2003;7:211–8.
27. Cowgill S, Gillman R, Kraemer E, et al. Ten-year follow-up after laparoscopic Nissen fundoplication for GERD. Am Surg 2007;73:748–52.
28. Terry M, Smith CD, Branum GD, et al. Outcomes of laparoscopic fundoplication for gastroesophageal reflux disease and paraesophageal hernia: experience with 1000 consecutive cases. Surg Endosc 2001;15:691–9.
29. Oelchalager BK, Quiroga E, Parra J, et al. Long-term outcomes after laparoscopic antireflux surgery. Am J Gastroenterol 2008;103:280–7.
30. Sandby R, Sundbom M. Nationwide survey of long-term results of laparoscopic antireflux surgery in Sweden. Scand J Gastroenterol 2010;45:15–20.
31. Roddenbery SA, Ross S, Morton C, et al. Laparoendoscopic single site (LESS) fundoplication: initial experience with safety and reduction of symptoms. J Gastrointet Surg, in press.
32. Galvani C, Fisichella PM, Gorodner MV, et al. Symptoms are a poor indicator of reflux status after fundoplication for gastroesophageal reflux disease: role of esophageal functions tests. Arch Surg 2003;138:514–9.

Achalasia

William C. Beck, MD, Kenneth W. Sharp, MD*

KEYWORDS

• Achalasia • Esophagomyotomy • Lower esophageal sphincter
• Esophageal motility

HISTORY

The history of achalasia dates back to 1679 when Sir Thomas Willis of Britain noted that some patients were not able to pass solid foods from the esophagus to the stomach. He was the first to devise a treatment for this disease, which involved a whale bone with an attached sponge that was used to push the food bolus from the esophagus into the stomach.[1] With this innovative new treatment, the patient lived for 15 years. Von Mikulicz named this phenomenon "cardiospasm" in 1882, and later described the performance of a lower esophageal dilation via a gastrotomy in 1904. In 1913, Ernest Heller performed the first esophagomyotomy for the treatment of cardiospasm, which involved both an anterior and posterior myotomy. The term achalasia, or "failure to relax," was promoted in 1924 by A.F. Hurst, who proposed that esophageal dilation was due to the absence of physiologic relaxation of the lower esophageal sphincter (LES) rather than an abnormal contraction.[2] In 1937, Frederick Lendrum published a paper supporting the notion that the "cardiospasm" term be changed, as he did not agree that esophageal dilation was due to the spasm of the LES. He reviewed 13 autopsy specimens obtained from patients with achalasia and noted that in all subjects the vagus nerve was intact and normal in structure, while there was noted to be a loss of ganglion cells in the myenteric plexus in all specimens reviewed.[3] These findings supported the proposal of Hurst, and cardiospasm began to be known as achalasia. The treatment of achalasia has undergone continued evolution, but mainstays of treatment continue to be predicated on dilation, myotomy, and more recently chemical paralysis of the LES.

DEFINITION AND PATHOPHYSIOLOGY

Achalasia is a chronic, incurable disease characterized by incomplete or absent relaxation of the LES and aperistalsis of the esophageal body. This condition results in

The authors have nothing to disclose.

Division of General Surgery, Department of Surgery, Vanderbilt University Medical Center, Vanderbilt University, 1161 Medical Center Drive, Room D-5203 MCN, Nashville, TN 37232-2577, USA
* Corresponding author.
E-mail address: ken.sharp@vanderbilt.edu

Surg Clin N Am 91 (2011) 1031–1037
doi:10.1016/j.suc.2011.06.005
surgical.theclinics.com
0039-6109/11/$ – see front matter © 2011 Elsevier Inc. All rights reserved.

difficulty taking liquid or solid food with resultant dilation of the esophagus. Esophageal tortuosity is seen in later stages of the disease if untreated. Achalasia is seen with equal frequency in men and women, and occurs in both children and the elderly, though the average age at diagnosis is in the sixth decade of life. Its incidence and prevalence was stated to be 1.63 per 100,000 and 10.82 per 100,000, respectively, in a recent North American study.[4]

The esophagus and LES are innervated by both inhibitory and excitatory neurons. The pathophysiology of achalasia is linked to the destruction of ganglion cells present in the esophageal wall and LES, which impairs the relaxation of the LES.[3] This destruction of ganglion cells is associated with an inflammatory response including lymphocytic infiltrates, which would seem to implicate an autoimmune, viral, or chronic degenerative process.[5] In a small minority of patients with Allgrove syndrome, a mutation on chromosome 12 is implicated in the development of achalasia. Pseudoachalasia, in which a functional distal esophageal obstruction mimics primary achalasia, is seen in patients with obstructing gastroesophageal junction tumors, Chagas disease, and amyloidosis. In addition, functional obstruction of the LES may also be caused following a fundoplication or gastric banding procedure. Pseudoachalasia is more likely in patients who undergo rapid weight loss or onset of dysphagia, as opposed to the more insidious onset of primary achalasia.

DIAGNOSIS

Patients with achalasia present with a history of dysphagia of solids and liquids. These patients often also have a history of weight loss, regurgitation of undigested food, and avoidance of certain solid foods that are difficult to swallow. About half of patients with achalasia will complain of chest pain or heartburn.[6] Some patients will complain of chest pain during or after eating that may be relieved with the emesis of undigested food. A history of aspiration and/or aspiration pneumonia may be elicited. When a patient presents with suspected achalasia, a barium swallow should be the first study performed, as up to 95% of patients with achalasia will have a positive barium swallow.[7] In a positive study, an aperistaltic esophagus is observed with tapering of the distal esophagus to the characteristic “bird’s beak” at the level of the esophageal hiatus. In addition, a dilated esophagus is usually seen, along with undigested food particles.[8,9] In patients with vigorous achalasia, repetitive nonperistaltic contractions may be visualized, classically associated with simultaneous high-pressure esophageal contractions.[10]

After a barium swallow has been performed, esophageal endoscopy should be performed to evaluate the patient for other causes of esophageal obstruction, such as esophageal cancer, which is known to be more prevalent in achalasia patients.[11] Endoscopic findings in patients with achalasia may include the presence of retained food particles or fluid in a dilated or tortuous esophagus.

Esophageal manometry is the key test for the diagnosis of esophageal achalasia. Manometry is performed with the patient in the supine position for the evaluation of LES function. In patients with achalasia, the lower esophageal resting pressure can be normal or elevated, with an elevated LES pressure being present about half the time.[12,13] The absence of any esophageal peristaltic contractions and the failure of the LES to relax to less than 8 mm Hg is diagnostic for achalasia.[12] Some variation of manometric results is noted in patients in patients with confirmed diagnoses of achalasia. Hirano and colleagues[14] describe 4 distinct variations of manometric measurements: (1) presence of high-amplitude esophageal body contractions, (2) short-segment esophageal body peristalsis, (3) retained complete deglutative LES relaxation, and (4) intact transient LES relaxation. Recently, the advent of esophageal topography in conjunction with high-resolution esophageal manometry has led to the development of the Chicago Classification of esophageal motility disorders.[15] Using esophageal topography, aperistalsis and the impaired relaxation at the level of the gastroesophageal junction is still seen in patients with achalasia. The ability to delineate the location of contractions is the strength of esophageal topography and may aid in the diagnosis of vigorous achalasia, in which spastic contractions are noted in the distal esophageal segment.

TREATMENT

Pharmacologic

The pharmacologic treatment of achalasia centers on inducing relaxation of the LES. Nitrates and calcium channel blockers (CCB) reduce the contraction of smooth muscle by increasing the concentration of cyclic guanosine monophosphate or decreasing the cellular uptake of calcium, respectively. Both nitrates and CCBs have been used to induce LES relaxation and reduce the amplitude of the esophageal peristaltic contractions. In a randomized, double-blind, placebo-controlled study Triadafilopoulos and colleagues[16] found that while both verapamil and nifedipine reduced the LES pressure at rest, no change in the LES deglutative relaxation was noted and improvement in symptoms was observed. Some improvement in individual patient complaints of heartburn was observed with both verapamil and nifedipine. Other studies have been published with similar manometric results, but also fail to induce total symptom resolution and incur high symptom recurrence rates.[17,18] Nitrates and CCBs are largely ineffective for the long-term treatment of achalasia, particularly when other currently available techniques are available with lower morbidity and higher rates of success.

Botulism toxin (BT) works by inhibiting the release of acetylcholine in muscle synapses and thereby inhibits the contraction of muscle. The first use of BT to inhibit the contraction of the LES was described in 1993 by Pasricha and colleagues.[19] BT is administered by injecting 80 to 100 units into 4 quadrants of the LES via an endoscopic delivery device. Multiple studies have been undertaken to evaluate the efficacy of BT injection for the treatment of achalasia. The treatment is effective for the resolution of symptoms at 1 month, with 78% to 90% of patients experiencing an improvement or resolution of their symptoms at 1 month.[20–26] At 1 year, however, symptomatic improvement was noted only in 35% to 41% of patients.[20,24] A recent trial combined the use of pneumatic dilation (PD) with intersphincteric BT injection. Of these patients 75% had either no symptoms or very mild symptoms 5 years following the combined treatment, but 20% of the original cohort was eventually referred for myotomy for recurrent dysphagia. The use of the combined modality was moderately effective for the treatment of achalasia, but not significantly better than PD alone. Given these findings, BT injection has a role in the treatment of achalasia for the high-risk patient or those patients with contraindications to PD or myotomy, but the high recurrence rate of BT injection makes surgical myotomy the treatment of choice for younger patients or those who do not have contraindications to surgical therapy.

Pneumatic Dilation

Dilation of the distal esophagus has been used in the treatment of achalasia since it was first recognized as a disease by Sir Thomas Willis.[1] The goal of PD is to disrupt the muscle fibers of the LES without causing full-thickness perforation, thereby facilitating the passage of the food bolus into the stomach. One of the first studies to report long-term follow-up of PD was published in 1971 by Vantrappen and colleagues.[27] These investigators noted a 77% "excellent" or "good" result in patients who were treated by serial PDs and followed for a minimum of 3 years following their last dilation. The perforation rate was approximately 1% with an overall complication rate of 11.3%. In modern series, the perforation rate associated with PD is 1% to 3%.[28,29] In randomized controlled trials, BT and PD were equally effective in relieving symptoms of achalasia immediately postprocedure, but patients treated with BT were more likely to recur at 12 months (87% vs 30%) as opposed to those treated with PD.[30,31] When multiple dilations are performed, long-term success rates (>12 months remission) are reported to be 60% to 85% in the achalasia cohort.[28,32] Predictors of failure of PD are young age at presentation, classic achalasia, elevated LES pressure at 3 months following dilation, and an incomplete expansion of the balloon at PD.[33] PD may be performed as an outpatient procedure, and patients are often able to quickly return to work following dilation. The observed complication rate associated with PD is low, but special consideration must be given to the possibility of perforation. Given these findings, LES PD is desirable in the treatment of high-risk operative patients, patients with failed myotomies, or patients who do not wish to undergo an operation, but is inferior to operative myotomy in the long-term relief of symptoms.

Esophageal Myotomy

Esophageal myotomy was initially performed by Ernest Heller in 1913 in an effort to relieve the distal esophageal obstruction that occurs with achalasia. He performed an anterior and posterior myotomy that extended 2 cm onto the stomach. Prior to 1991, the esophageal myotomy was routinely performed via a thoracic approach, but this technique often made it difficult to carry the myotomy far enough onto the stomach to be effective and also carried the morbidity of a thoracotomy. Many early failures of myotomy for achalasia were attributable to an incomplete myotomy.[34] A complete esophagomyotomy involves the division of the LES for 5 to 8 cm on the distal aspect of the esophagus, with the continuation of the myotomy for 2 cm onto the stomach.[35–37] On the completion of the myotomy, the esophageal mucosa is seen to be bulging from between the muscle edges. In 1991, Shimi and colleagues[38] described a laparoscopic approach for performing an anterior esophagomyotomy in patients with achalasia. A subsequent study in 1997 outlining the performance of laparoscopic Heller myotomy (LHM) describes resolution of symptoms in 90% of patients.[39] In 1999, Patti and colleagues[35] reported a group of 168 patients who underwent thoracoscopic myotomy or LHM with fundoplication. There were no observed mortalities. The incidence of gastroesophageal reflux was postoperatively 17% versus 60% in the subsets of patients who underwent LHM versus thoracoscopic myotomy. In addition, the length of stay was 24 hours shorter, and the symptoms of dysphagia were more successfully relieved in the laparoscopic group (85% vs 93%). LHM also eliminates or reduces the symptoms of chest pain in patients with achalasia.[40] With these results, LHM became the standard of care for the operative treatment in patients with achalasia, and similar high success rates with very low morbidity have been repeatedly reported.[41] Rates of postoperative perforation and mortality are consistently lower than those for contemporary series of PD.

The type of fundoplication performed in conjunction with the Heller myotomy remains a topic of much debate. In comparison with the treatment of reflux disease whereby peristalsis is normal, achalasia patients may not generate enough force to adequately propel the food bolus through a 360° wrap. Numerous randomized controlled trials have been performed to evaluate the effectiveness of partial fundoplications in preventing reflux following esophagomyotomy. In a comparison prospective, randomized, controlled, blinded clinical trial, Heller myotomy with Dor (anterior) fundoplication reduced the postoperative incidence of reflux by 39% (48% vs 9%).[36] A subsequent trial of LHM with Dor fundoplication versus LHM with Nissen fundoplication found that both techniques were sufficient and effective in controlling postoperative reflux, but the subset of patients who underwent Nissen fundoplication experienced a 15% rate of postoperative dysphagia compared with 3% in the Dor group.[42] A Dor fundoplication is also preferred in cases of intraoperative esophageal perforation as a method to buttress the esophageal mucosal defect.[34] Patients undergoing LHM with Toupet (posterior) fundoplication experienced a 33% rate of postoperative reflux among those patients diagnosed by pH studies. The Toupet fundoplication is favored by some surgeons over the anterior fundoplication, but prospective comparison of the two techniques has not been performed and the choice of fundoplication is based on surgeon preference. Based on this information, a partial fundoplication should be performed in conjunction with LHM when technical factors permit. However, long-term follow-up studies of a large number of patients undergoing partial fundoplication with Heller myotomy have not been performed.

SUMMARY

Achalasia is a rare esophageal motility disorder that is characterized by absent peristalsis and failure of the LES to relax, thereby preventing the normal passage of solids and liquids into the stomach caused by a destruction of the ganglionic neurons within the esophageal muscularis and LES. Management of achalasia with sublingual nitrates or CCBs is not recommended, due to the high failure rates and poorly tolerated side effects, except in patients who cannot tolerate other treatment modalities. Injection of the LES with BT is effective for short-term relief of dysphagia symptoms, but the effects are short lived and require frequent reinterventions to maintain efficacy. PD of the LES is moderately effective for the relief of dysphagia in the short and intermediate term, but often requires repeat dilations and carries a small but significant risk of esophageal perforation. Dilation remains a valuable option for those high-risk patients in whom operative intervention carries too high a risk or in whom Heller myotomy has failed. With the advent of minimally invasive Heller myotomy and its incumbent low morbidity and mortality rates, an LHM with partial fundoplication is a durable, safe, and effective treatment option for patients with achalasia.

REFERENCES

1. Brewer LA 3rd. History of surgery of the esophagus. Am J Surg 1980;139(6): 730–43.
2. Hurst AF, Rowlands RP. Case of achalasia of the cardia relieved by operation. Proc R Soc Med 1924;17:45–6.
3. Lendrum F. Anatomic features of the cardiac orifice of the stomach with special reference to cardiospasm. Arch Intern Med 1937;59:474–511.
4. Sadowski DC, Ackah F, Jiang B, et al. Achalasia: incidence, prevalence and survival. A population-based study. Neurogastroenterol Motil 2010;22(9): e256–61.
5. Farrokhi F, Vaezi MF. Idiopathic (primary) achalasia. Orphanet J Rare Dis 2007;2:38.
6. Spechler SJ, Souza RF, Rosenberg SJ, et al. Heartburn in patients with achalasia. Gut 1995;37(3):305–8.
7. Ott DJ, Richter JE, Chen YM, et al. Esophageal radiography and manometry: correlation in 172 patients with dysphagia. AJR Am J Roentgenol 1987;149(2): 307–11.

8. Margulis AR, Koehler RE. Radiologic diagnosis of disordered esophageal motility: a unified physiologic approach. Radiol Clin North Am 1976;14(3): 429–39.
9. Stewart ET. Radiographic evaluation of the esophagus and its motor disorders. Med Clin North Am 1981;65(6):1173–94.
10. Summerton SL. Radiographic evaluation of esophageal function. Gastrointest Endosc Clin N Am 2005;15(2):231–42.
11. Sandler RS, Nyren O, Ekbom A, et al. The risk of esophageal cancer in patients with achalasia. A population-based study. JAMA 1995;274(17):1359–62.
12. Gideon RM. Manometry: technical issues. Gastrointest Endosc Clin N Am 2005; 15(2):243–55.
13. Fisichella PM, Raz D, Palazzo F, et al. Clinical, radiological, and manometric profile in 145 patients with untreated achalasia. World J Surg 2008;32(9):1974–9.
14. Hirano I, Tatum RP, Shi G, et al. Manometric heterogeneity in patients with idiopathic achalasia. Gastroenterology 2001;120(4):789–98.
15. Kahrilas PJ, Ghosh SK, Pandolfino JE. Esophageal motility disorders in terms of pressure topography: the Chicago Classification. J Clin Gastroenterol 2008;42(5): 627–35.
16. Triadafilopoulos G, Aaronson M, Sackel S, et al. Medical treatment of esophageal achalasia. Double-blind crossover study with oral nifedipine, verapamil, and placebo. Dig Dis Sci 1991;36(3):260–7.
17. Gelfond M, Rozen P, Gilat T. Isosorbide dinitrate and nifedipine treatment of achalasia: a clinical, manometric and radionuclide evaluation. Gastroenterology 1982; 83(5):963–9.
18. Traube M, Dubovik S, Lange RC, et al. The role of nifedipine therapy in achalasia: results of a randomized, double-blind, placebo-controlled study. Am J Gastroenterol 1989;84(10):1259–62.
19. Pasricha PJ, Ravich WJ, Kalloo AN. Botulinum toxin for achalasia. Lancet 1993; 341(8839):244–5.
20. Annese V, D'Onofrio V, Andriulli A. Botulinum toxin in long-term therapy for achalasia. Ann Intern Med 1998;128(8):696.
21. Annese V, Basciani M, Borrelli O, et al. Intrasphincteric injection of botulinum toxin is effective in long-term treatment of esophageal achalasia. Muscle Nerve 1998; 21(11):1540–2.
22. Annese V, Bassotti G, Coccia G, et al. Comparison of two different formulations of botulinum toxin A for the treatment of oesophageal achalasia. The Gismad Achalasia Study Group. Aliment Pharmacol Ther 1999;13(10):1347–50.
23. Annese V, Bassotti G, Coccia G, et al. A multicentre randomised study of intrasphincteric botulinum toxin in patients with oesophageal achalasia. GISMAD Achalasia Study Group. Gut 2000;46(5):597–600.
24. Martinek J, Siroky M, Plottova Z, et al. Treatment of patients with achalasia with botulinum toxin: a multicenter prospective cohort study. Dis Esophagus 2003; 16(3):204–9.
25. Pasricha PJ, Rai R, Ravich WJ, et al. Botulinum toxin for achalasia: long-term outcome and predictors of response. Gastroenterology 1996;110(5):1410–5.
26. Cuilliere C, Ducrotte P, Zerbib F, et al. Achalasia: outcome of patients treated with intrasphincteric injection of botulinum toxin. Gut 1997;41(1):87–92.
27. Vantrappen G, Hellemans J, Deloof W, et al. Treatment of achalasia with pneumatic dilatations. Gut 1971;12(4):268–75.
28. Katz PO, Gilbert J, Castell DO. Pneumatic dilatation is effective long-term treatment for achalasia. Dig Dis Sci 1998;43(9):1973–7.

29. Kadakia SC, Wong RK. Pneumatic balloon dilation for esophageal achalasia. Gastrointest Endosc Clin N Am 2001;11(2):325–46, vii.
30. Ghoshal UC, Chaudhuri S, Pal BB, et al. Randomized controlled trial of intra-sphincteric botulinum toxin A injection versus balloon dilatation in treatment of achalasia cardia. Dis Esophagus 2001;14(3–4):227–31.
31. Mikaeli J, Fazel A, Montazeri G, et al. Randomized controlled trial comparing botulinum toxin injection to pneumatic dilatation for the treatment of achalasia. Aliment Pharmacol Ther 2001;15(9):1389–96.
32. Eckardt VF, Aignherr C, Bernhard G. Predictors of outcome in patients with achalasia treated by pneumatic dilation. Gastroenterology 1992;103(6):1732–8.
33. Alderliesten J, Conchillo JM, Leeuwenburgh I, et al. Predictors for outcome of failure of balloon dilatation in patients with achalasia. Gut 2011;60(1):10–6.
34. Sharp KW, Khaitan L, Scholz S, et al. 100 consecutive minimally invasive Heller myotomies: lessons learned. Ann Surg 2002;235(5):631–8 [discussion: 638–9].
35. Patti MG, Pellegrini CA, Horgan S, et al. Minimally invasive surgery for achalasia: an 8-year experience with 168 patients. Ann Surg 1999;230(4):587–93 [discussion: 593–584].
36. Richards WO, Torquati A, Holzman MD, et al. Heller myotomy versus Heller myotomy with Dor fundoplication for achalasia: a prospective randomized double-blind clinical trial. Ann Surg 2004;240(3):405–12 [discussion: 412–405].
37. Tatum RP, Pellegrini CA. How I do it: laparoscopic Heller myotomy with Toupet fundoplication for achalasia. J Gastrointest Surg 2009;13(6):1120–4.
38. Shimi S, Nathanson LK, Cuschieri A. Laparoscopic cardiomyotomy for achalasia. J R Coll Surg Edinb 1991;36(3):152–4.
39. Hunter JG, Trus TL, Branum GD, et al. Laparoscopic Heller myotomy and fundoplication for achalasia. Ann Surg 1997;225(6):655–64 [discussion: 664–655].
40. Omura N, Kashiwagi H, Yano F, et al. Effect of laparoscopic esophagomyotomy on chest pain associated with achalasia and prediction of therapeutic outcomes. Surg Endosc 2011;25:1048–53.
41. Zaninotto G, Costantini M, Rizzetto C, et al. Four hundred laparoscopic myotomies for esophageal achalasia: a single centre experience. Ann Surg 2008; 248(6):986–93.
42. Rebecchi F, Giaccone C, Farinella E, et al. Randomized controlled trial of laparoscopic Heller myotomy plus Dor fundoplication versus Nissen fundoplication for achalasia: long-term results. Ann Surg 2008;248(6):1023–30.

Gastric Adenocarcinoma Surgery and Adjuvant Therapy

Sameer H. Patel, MD, David A. Kooby, MD*

KEYWORDS

- Gastric cancer • Gastric resection • Adjuvant therapy
- Gastric adenocarcinoma

Although the incidence of gastric cancer in the United States has steadily declined since the 1930s, globally it remains the second leading cause of cancer-related mortality.[1] This ominous diagnosis affected approximately 21,000 individuals in the United States in 2010 and, despite existing treatments, an estimated 10,570 (50%) of those patients succumbed to the disease.[2] The incidence of gastric cancer varies substantially worldwide, with the highest rates (>20 per 100,000) occurring in Japan, China, eastern Europe, and South America.[1] By contrast, the lowest rates (<10 per 100,000) are found in North America, southern Asia, North and East Africa, Australia, and New Zealand.[1] Gastric cancer is also more common in men than in women (10.9 vs 5.5 per 100,000) and more common in African American, Asian, Hispanic, and Native American people.[3] Prognosis for all races has significantly improved since 1975; 5-year survival improved from 16% to 27% in 2005.[2] The term gastric cancer is broad, applying to multiple malignancies of varying histology. Specifically, it can include adenocarcinoma, lymphoma, gastrointestinal stromal tumors (GIST), squamous cell carcinoma, carcinoid tumors, and adenoacanthoma. Adenocarcinoma accounts for more than 90% of gastric malignancies and is the focus of this review.

CLASSIFICATION OF GASTRIC CANCER

The primary histopathologic classification used for gastric cancer was first described in 1965 by Lauren.[4] This system divides gastric adenocarcinomas into 2 types: diffuse gastric adenocarcinomas (DGCA) and intestinal gastric adenocarcinomas (IGCA) (**Table 1**).[4] DGCA develops in younger patients, with similar incidences among men

---

This work has no funding, and the authors have nothing to disclose.
Division of Surgical Oncology, Department of Surgery, Winship Cancer Institute, Emory University, 1365C Clifton Road, Northeast 2nd Floor, Atlanta, GA 30322, USA
* Corresponding author.
E-mail address: dkooby@emory.edu

Surg Clin N Am 91 (2011) 1039–1077
doi:10.1016/j.suc.2011.06.009
surgical.theclinics.com
0039-6109/11/$ – see front matter © 2011 Elsevier Inc. All rights reserved.

Table 1
Laurén classification of gastric cancer

Variable	Intestinal Type	Diffuse Type
Age	Older population	Younger population
Sex	Male/female ratio 2:1	Male ≈ female
Association	Environmental factors	Hereditary
Preexisting factors	Associated with atrophic gastritis	Associated with blood type A
Symptoms	Well-differentiated glands, intestinal metaplasia	Poorly differentiated, signet ring cells
Location in stomach	Antrum (distal)	Corpus, fundus (proximal)
Pattern of spread	Hematogenous	Lymphatic and transmural
Metastasis	Liver metastasis	Peritoneal metastasis
World Health Organization equivalent	Papillary, tubular, mucinous, poorly differentiated	Poorly differentiated, signet ring cell
Japanese equivalent	Differentiated type	Poorly differentiated type

Data from Vauhkonen M, Vauhkonen H, Sipponen P. Pathology and molecular biology of gastric cancer. Best Pract Res Clin Gastroenterol 2006;20(4):651–74; and Munson JL, O'Mahony R. Radical gastrectomy for cancer of the stomach. Surg Clin North Am 2005;85(5):1021–32, vii.

and women, and spreads by direct tumor extension often resulting in peritoneal metastasis. Submucosal infiltrative growth is also a characteristic of DGCA, occasionally resulting in a rigid, thickened, leather-bottle appearance of the stomach, called linitis plastica (found in 12%–14% of advanced gastric cancers).[5] IGCA arises in the older population with increased incidence in men. It is common in endemic areas, associated with environmental factors, atrophic gastritis, and spreads hematogenously, often resulting in liver metastasis. Because of the importance of inflammation and environmental factors in the development of IGCA, Correa and colleagues[6] proposed a multistep progression from *Helicobacter pylori* infection and gastritis to IGCA.[7] This model only applies to IGCA and does not explain the progression of DGCA, suggesting that the diffuse and intestinal types have a unique molecular and pathologic biology. Other known risk factors associated with the development of gastric cancer are listed in **Box 1**.[8]

On pathologic examination, DGCA microscopically appears as a mass of mucocellular cells with poor glandular differentiation, whereas the intestinal type have well-formed glands or branching tubular structures.[9,10] Grossly, DGCA appear as ulcers on endoscopy, whereas intestinal types appear as exophytic, bulky lesions.[9,10]

Several other classification systems exist; however, none are able to reliably predict survival. Thus far, the clinical stage of gastric cancer, provided by the American Joint Cancer Commission (AJCC), is the single most important prognostic factor for survival (**Table 2**).[9]

HEREDITARY GASTRIC CANCER

Although most gastric cancers arise sporadically, 1% to 3% are hereditary in nature.[11–13] The most common type of familial gastric cancer is hereditary diffuse gastric cancer (HDGC).[14] HDGC is characterized by an autosomal dominant inheritance pattern with greater than 80% penetrance and diffuse signet ring cells.[15] Based on the International Gastric Cancer Linkage Consortium, a family is diagnosed with HDGC if they meet the following criteria:

Box 1
Risk factors associated with the development of gastric cancer

- *H pylori* gastric infection
- Advanced age
- Male gender
- Race: Hispanic Americans, African Americans, Asian/Pacific Islanders
- Diet low in fruits and vegetables
- Diet high in salted, smoked, or preserved foods
- Obesity
- Chronic atrophic gastritis
- Intestinal metaplasia
- Pernicious anemia
- Gastric adenomatous polyps
- Family history of gastric cancer
- Cigarette smoking
- Menetrier disease (giant hypertrophic gastritis)
- Familial adenomatous polyposis
- Certain occupations (coal, metal, and rubber industries)

Data from Gastric Cancer Treatment (PDQ) 2010. Available at: http://www.cancer.gov/cancertopics/pdq/treatment/gastric/. Accessed December 28, 2010.

1. Two or more documented cases of diffuse gastric cancer in first-degree or second-degree relatives, with at least 1 diagnosed before the age of 50 years, or
2. Three or more cases of documented diffuse gastric cancer in first-degree/second-degree relatives, independent of age of onset[14,15]

In 1998 Guilford and colleagues[16] examined the presence of an early onset, poorly differentiated, high-grade, diffuse gastric cancer in a large kindred of Maori in New Zealand. Genetic analysis revealed that a germline mutation of the tumor suppressor gene, E-cadherin (CDH1), was the basis behind HDGC in this group of people. Further studies have revealed that approximately 25% to 40% of families meeting the criteria for HDGC have a mutation in the CDH1 gene.[14,15,17] There are a variety of mutations that can arise in CDH1, including truncations (75%–80%) and missense mutations (20%–25%).[15,18] In sporadic gastric cancer, mutations in CDH1 do occur but are often clustered around exons 7 and 8; however, in the familial type, the germline mutations can span the entire gene (16 exons).[15] Mutations in CDH1 can be detected using multiplex ligation–dependent probe amplification (MLPA) or array-comparative genomic hybridization (CGH) and, after confirmation, genetic counseling is mandatory. Testing for family members with HDGC usually begins in the late teens or 20s, and asymptomatic carriers of mutations are offered prophylactic total gastrectomy with Roux-en-Y reconstruction.[14] There is no absolute age at which patients who are positive for the CDH1 mutant should undergo surgery; however, total gastrectomy is recommended in any CDH1-positive patient with a positive biopsy and/or age greater than 20 years.[14,18] For patients who do not choose to undergo prophylactic gastrectomy, annual surveillance endoscopy should be performed until the patient is ready to

Table 2
AJCC 7th edition tumor-node-metastasis (TNM) classification and staging of gastric cancer

Primary Tumor (T)	
TX	Primary tumor cannot be assessed
T0	No evidence of primary tumor
Tis	Carcinoma in situ: intraepithelial tumor without invasion of the lamina propria
T1	Tumor invades lamina propria or muscularis mucosae, or submucosa
T1a	Tumor invades lamina propria or muscularis mucosae
T1b	Tumor invades submucosa
T2	Tumor invades muscularis propria
T3	Tumor penetrates subserosal connective tissue without invasion of visceral peritoneum or adjacent structures. T3 tumors also include those extending into the gastrocolic or gastrohepatic ligaments, or into the greater or lesser omentum, without perforation of the visceral peritoneum covering these structures
T4	Tumor invades serosa (visceral peritoneum) or adjacent structures
T4a	Tumor invades serosa (visceral peritoneum)
T4b	Tumor invades adjacent structures such as spleen, transverse colon, liver, diaphragm, pancreas, abdominal wall, adrenal gland, kidney, small intestine, and retroperitoneum
Lymph Nodes (N)	
NX	Regional lymph node(s) cannot be assessed
N0	No regional lymph node metastasis
N1	Metastasis in 1–2 regional lymph nodes
N2	Metastasis in 3–6 regional lymph nodes
N3	Metastasis in ≥7 regional lymph nodes
Metastasis (M)	
MX	Distant metastasis cannot be assessed
M0	No distant metastasis
M1	Distant metastasis (including positive peritoneal cytology)

Staging	T	N	M	5-y survival (%)
Stage 0	Tis	N0	M0	—
Stage IA	T1	N0	M0	70.8
Stage IB	T2	N0	M0	57.4
	T1	N1	M0	—
Stage IIA	T3	N0	M0	45.5
	T2	N1	M0	—
	T1	N2	M0	—
Stage IIB	T4a	N0	M0	32.8
	T3	N1	M0	—
	T2	N2	M0	—
	T1	N3	M0	—
Stage IIIA	T4a	N1	M0	19.8
	T3	N2	M0	—
	T2	N3	M0	—
Stage IIIB	T4b	N0 or N1	M0	14.0
	T4a	N2	M0	—
	T3	N3	M0	—
Stage IIIC	T4b	N2 or N3	M0	9.2
	T4a	N3	M0	—
Stage IV	Any T	Any N	M1	4.0

Data from Washington K. 7th edition of the AJCC cancer staging manual: stomach. Ann Surg Oncol 2010;17(12):3077–9.

proceed based on genetic risk alone. Because of the significant physical as well as psychological impact of performing a total gastrectomy in a young patient, a multidisciplinary team approach is compulsory.

Mutations in CDH1 also place patients at an increased risk of developing lobular breast cancer and colon cancer with signet ring cell features.[14] Therefore, early breast cancer and colon cancer screening should also be performed in these family members.

CLINICAL MANIFESTATIONS

Most patients diagnosed with gastric cancer present with advanced stages of disease because early symptoms are often nonspecific. The most common symptoms at time of presentation are weight loss (40%) secondary to anorexia and vague abdominal pain (58%).[19] Symptoms also vary based on location of the primary lesion. For proximal tumors involving the gastroesophageal junction, dysphagia is common. By contrast, distal or antral tumors often result in nausea and vomiting, and carry a higher risk of gastric outlet obstruction. With diffuse, infiltrative disease, such as linitis plastica, in which the stomach wall is thickened and rigid, patients often develop early satiety. Chronic anemia is another common finding (40%) often manifesting as iron deficiency anemia in patients with heme-positive stool; however, frank gastrointestinal bleeding with hematemesis is rare (5%).

Traditional physical examination findings are most often seen with metastatic or locally advanced disease and are reflective of the pattern of spread. Patients who present with a palpable abdominal mass typically have a large, locally advanced tumor. Hematogenous metastases to the liver may result in jaundice, ascites, or hepatomegaly. Lymphatic spread can lead to a palpable left supraclavicular (Virchow node) or periumbilical lymph node (Sister Mary Joseph node). Peritoneal metastasis may be identified as a palpable ovarian mass (Krukenberg tumor) on pelvic examination, or as an extraluminal mass on rectal examination (Blumer shelf). Other nonspecific cutaneous findings include acanthosis nigricans and eruption of multiple seborrheic keratoses (sign of Leser-Trélat).[20] Studies examining the pattern of metastasis suggest that peritoneal disease is associated with DGCA, younger patients, poor differentiation, and signet ring cell histology.[21,22] Hepatic metastases are more common with IGCA and well-differentiated to moderately differentiated histologies.[21,22] Regardless of site, organ failure from metastatic lesions is the most common cause of death for patients with advanced gastric cancer.

DIAGNOSIS AND STAGING OF GASTRIC CANCER

The diagnosis of early gastric cancer varies substantially between the Western world and the East, where early, intense screening is standard. Incidence rates (per 100,000) vary from 10.9 in men and 5.0 in women in the United States to 65.9 in men and 25.9 in women in Korea.[3,23] Countries with the highest incidences of gastric cancer are Korea, Japan, China, Belarus, Costa Rica, and Russia.[23] In Japan, approximately 50% of gastric tumors are diagnosed early; by contrast, only 5% to 10% of cases in the United States are diagnosed early.[24,25] In the West, 5-year overall survival (OS) is a dismal 20%, whereas it is considerably better in the East, as a result of aggressive screening. Ahn and colleagues[26] reviewed their single-institution data from Seoul, Korea between 1986 and 2006, examining clinicopathologic features and survival data. Of their 12,026 patients who had gastric cancer and who underwent gastrectomy, 5-year survival was 73.2%.

Although the global incidence of gastric cancer overall is decreasing, there has been a shift in the relative locations of the lesions within the stomach. In the United States, many European countries, and Asia, the incidence of gastric cancers within the cardia and proximal stomach have increased, whereas lesions in the fundus and distal stomach have decreased.[23,27,28] El-Serag[29] proposed that the rising incidence of gastroesophageal reflux disease in the obese population has resulted in the increase of proximal gastric cancers.

Initial investigation for gastric cancer should begin with a thorough history and physical examination. The history should focus on questions pertaining to the risk factors mentioned in **Box 1** and physical examination findings to detect any skin changes or palpable masses, which often indicate advanced or metastatic disease.

Basic laboratory investigations should include complete blood cell count to check for anemia, metabolic panels to evaluate electrolyte abnormalities associated with possible gastric outlet obstruction, and liver enzymes for possible metastasis. Certain tumor markers have also been shown to be prognostic of poor outcome and aggressive disease. Higher levels of serum tumor markers, such as carcinoembryonic antigen (CEA), carbohydrate antigen (CA 19-9), and α-fetoprotein (AFP), correlate with depth of tumor invasion, pathologic stage, presence of vascular invasion, and liver and lymph node metastases.[30–34]

Gastric cancer screening is justified for patients in high-risk groups (see **Box 1**) and for those living in high-incidence areas.[35] In Japan, double-contrast barium meal studies and endoscopy are used.[36] Suzuki and colleagues[37] found that, of 1226 consecutive patients diagnosed with gastric cancer, 41.8% were symptomatic, and 91.6% of those patients went directly to endoscopy as opposed to barium study. For the 58.2% who were asymptomatic, 67.8% went directly to endoscopy and 32.2% went to barium study; thus, most patients, whether symptomatic or not, bypass barium studies and go straight to endoscopy for evaluation.[37]

Following diagnosis, staging commences with axial imaging, and computed tomography (CT) remains the modality of choice for this purpose. The sensitivity of a CT scan to determine nodal status ranges from 50% to 95% and specificity from 40% to 99%.[38–40] Magnetic resonance imaging (MRI) is slightly inferior to CT for nodal staging (55%–65% vs 59%–73%, $P>.05$).[41–43] Several studies suggest that MRI may improve detection of metastatic disease compared with CT, especially when the contrast ferumoxtran-10 is used (sensitivity 100%, specificity 92.6%).[41–44] 18F-fluoro-2-deoxyglucose positron emission tomography (FDG-PET) is increasingly used and can provide additional staging information, especially for metastatic disease; however, it is inferior to CT and MRI for screening (sensitivity 10.0%, specificity 99.2%).[45] For assessing depth of invasion, endoscopic ultrasonography (EUS) remains the primary choice for determining T staging.[46–49]

A large systematic review examining 31 studies conducted by Kwee and Kwee[50] evaluated the usefulness of using abdominal ultrasonography (AUS), EUS, multidetector computed tomography (MDCT), MRI, FDG-PET, and FDG-PET/CT fusion in assessing lymph node status in gastric cancer. They found that there was no imaging modality that consistently achieved both high sensitivity and high specificity in the detection of lymph node metastasis. Despite these disappointing findings, it is necessary to determine the extent of disease so that the appropriate surgical resection can take place.

It is the authors' practice to use EUS selectively to assess the depth of invasion (T staging) and regional node involvement (N staging) when the tumor is small, and the information guides the treatment approach. CT is preferred, rather than MRI, for staging, and FDG-PET is selectively used as an adjunct if there is high suspicion of distant metastatic disease in higher risk patients.

NODAL STAGING

The current AJCC tumor-node-metastasis (TNM) staging classification remains the best prognostic system for assessing survival from gastric adenocarcinoma (see **Table 2**). In 1997, nodal classification changed from using the location of the involved lymph nodes to the number (pN1, 1–6 nodes; pN2, 7–15 nodes; pN3, >15 nodes). For an adequate sampling, 15 lymph nodes need to be removed to accurately differentiate between pN2 and pN3 disease. However, several studies confirmed that the average number of nodes evaluated is close to 10, and that only about 30% of patients have at least 15 nodes evaluated.[51–53] This is an issue of both adequate dissection and thorough pathologic assessment. As a result of the routine inadequate nodal evaluation, the N stage was further modified. In the revised seventh edition of the AJCC staging, a minimum of 7 nodes are needed, and this is today's current classification system (pN1, 1–2 nodes; pN2, 3–6 nodes; pN3, ≥7 nodes).

More recent studies propose examining the metastatic lymph node ratio (MLR; the ratio between metastatic lymph nodes and total evaluated lymph nodes) as opposed to the total number of positive nodes. Autopsy studies have shown that, on average, D1 dissections can provide an average of 15 nodes, D2 dissections can produce 27 nodes, and 42 nodes may come from a D3 dissection.[54] MLR may be more valuable in cases in which inadequate node evaluation has been performed. Several groups have found MLR to be one of the strongest negative prognostic factors for survival on multivariate analyses, whereas AJCC N staging was not (MLR≤20%: hazard ratio [HR] 3.6, 95% confidence interval [CI] 1.2–11.2, $P = .025$. MLR>20%: HR 4.5, 95% CI 2.2–9.5, $P \leq .0001$).[55–57] This suggests that MLR may have greater prognostic value that N-staging alone. However, most of these studies had few patients with less than 15 nodes recovered, which would be the group to derive the greatest usefulness from MLR as opposed to the total number of positive nodes.[55–57] Additional studies are needed; nonetheless, MLR does show promise as an important prognostic marker and could potentially be added to the staging classification of gastric cancer in the future.

The Japanese Research Society for Gastric Cancer (JRSGC) established a different classification system for nodal metastasis. Like the original AJCC staging system, they use the anatomic location of the nodes, which are designated by stations (**Fig. 1**, **Table 3**).[58] Based on the stations involved, they are assigned into groups N1, N2, or N3 (see **Table 3**), and this corresponds with the degree of nodal dissection (removal of N1 nodes is a D1 dissection, removal of N2 nodes is D2 dissection, and removal of N3 nodes is D3 dissection). Given the sophistication of surgical dissection and pathologic analysis in Japan, and the frequency of gastric cancer, this regional nodal staging system works for them, but is not practical in the West.

PERITONEAL CYTOLOGY

Gastric cancer is notorious for its high recurrence rate after resection and for its ability to metastasize throughout the body via multiple pathways. In Japan, extensive lymphadenectomy during resection (D2–3) is used to provide better locoregional control. The failures that occur following extensive dissection are likely caused by peritoneal carcinomatosis.[59] Certain factors have been found to be associated with peritoneal recurrence, such as serosal involvement, younger patient age, diffuse histotype, and presence of infiltrative disease.[60,61] Sampling peritoneal washings for cytologic detection of malignant cells was incorporated into the Japanese staging system in 1998. Justification was provided by multiple studies that revealed that positive cytology was associated with peritoneal dissemination and was an independent

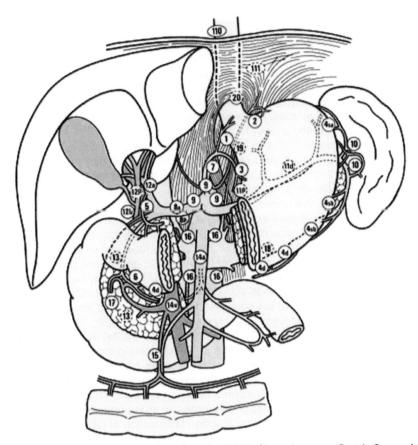

Fig. 1. Location of nodal stations based on the JRSGC. (*From* Japanese Gastric Cancer Association. Japanese classification of gastric carcinoma - 2nd English edition. Gastric Cancer 1998;1:16; with permission.)

prognostic factor of poor outcome.[61–66] A patient with positive cytology is classified as having stage IV disease.[58] In addition, positive cytology is associated with higher T stages and nodal involvement, and is one of the most accurate preoperative staging tools available.[67,68]

Bentrem and colleagues[69] investigated the predictive role of peritoneal cytology in patients undergoing curative resection for gastric cancer. They found that not only was positive preoperative cytology a significant predictor of outcome, along with site, T, and N staging, but it was the strongest predictor of death from gastric cancer (rate ratio 2.7, $P<.001$). With the most recent change in the AJCC criteria, the United States has adopted the Japanese system; positive peritoneal cytology is metastatic (M1) and, consequently, stage IV disease.[70] Therefore, staging laparoscopy with peritoneal cytology before resection is part of the initial workup and can potentially spare the patient a needless laparotomy in some cases. The investigators recommend obtaining staging laparoscopy and peritoneal washings, when possible, before instituting preoperative chemotherapy in higher risk patients (those with reduced performance status, proximal tumors, and those who are symptomatic from their disease).

Table 3
Lymph node station numbers based on the JRSGC

Station No.	Description	Location of Primary Tumor In Stomach: Upper one-third	Middle one-third	Lower one-third
No. 1	Right paracardial LN	1	1	2
No. 2	Left paracardial LN	1	3	M
No. 3	LN along the lesser curvature	1	1	1
No. 4sa	LN along the short gastric vessels	1	3	M
No. 4sb	LN along the left gastroepiploic vessels	1	1	3
No. 4d	LN along the right gastroepiploic vessels	2	1	1
No. 5	Suprapyloric LN	3	1	1
No. 6	Infrapyloric LN	3	1	1
No. 7	LN along the left gastric artery	2	2	2
No. 8a	LN along the common hepatic artery (anterosuperior group)	2	2	2
No. 8p	LN along the common hepatic artery (posterior group)	3	3	3
No. 9	LN around the celiac artery	2	2	2
No. 10	LN at the splenic hilum	2	3	M
No. 11p	LN along the proximal splenic artery	2	2	2
No. 11d	LN along the distal splenic artery	2	3	M
No. 12a	LN in the hepatoduodenal ligament (along the hepatic artery)	3	2	2
No. 12b	LN in the hepatoduodenal ligament (along the bile duct)	3	3	3
No. 12p	LN in the hepatoduodenal ligament (behind the portal vein)	3	3	3
No. 13	LN on the posterior surface of the pancreatic head	M	3	3
No. 14v	LN along the superior mesenteric vein	M	3	2
No. 14a	LN along the superior mesenteric artery	M	M	M
No. 15	LN along the middle colic vessels	M	M	M
No. 16a1	LN in the aortic hiatus	3	M	M
No. 16a2	LN around the abdominal aorta (from the upper margin of celiac trunk to the lower margin of the left renal vein)	M	3	3
No. 16b1	LN around abdominal aorta (from lower margin of the left renal vein to the upper margin of the inferior mesenteric artery)	M	3	3
No. 16b2	LN around the abdominal aorta (from the upper margin of inferior mesenteric artery to the aortic bifurcation)	M	M	M
No. 17	LN on the anterior surface of the pancreatic head	M	M	M
No. 18	LN along the inferior margin of the pancreas	M	M	M
No. 19	Infradiaphragmatic LN	3	M	M

(continued on next page)

Table 3
(continued)

Station No.	Description	Location of Primary Tumor In Stomach: Upper one-third	Middle one-third	Lower one-third
No. 20	LN in the esophageal hiatus of the diaphragm	3	M	M
No. 110	Paraesophageal LN in the lower thorax	M	M	M
No. 111	Supradiaphragmatic LN	M	M	M
No. 112	Posterior mediastinal LN	M	M	M

Extent of Node Metastasis	
N0:	No evidence of LN metastasis
N1:	Metastasis to Group 1 LNs, but no metastasis to Groups 2 or 3 LNs
N2:	Metastasis to Group 2 LNs, but no metastasis to Group 3 LNs
N3:	Metastasis to Group 3 LNs
NX:	Unknown

Abbreviations: LN, lymph node; M, lymph nodes considered distant metastasis.

SENTINEL LYMPH NODE BIOPSY

Lymph node status is one of the most important independent predictors of survival in gastric cancer. Sentinel lymph node biopsy (SLNbx) is routinely used in other malignances, such as breast cancer and melanoma, to determine whether more formal node dissection is necessary to adequately stage patients. Because much of the morbidity from gastric cancer surgery relates to lymphadenectomy, there is interest in perfecting this technique. For the procedure, a dye or radioactive tracer is injected in or near the tumor and the first draining nodal basin is identified visually or by the use of a γ probe. SLNbx can allow pathologists to perform more thorough analyses of index lymph nodes with more serial sections. This procedure, in turn, can guide the extent of further nodal dissection and therapy.

There is substantial variability in the techniques used for SLNbx. The procedure can be done endoscopically or during the open operation. Site of injection can be within the submucosa or subserosa. The dye or tracer used can be 2% patent blue dye, 1% isosulfan blue, technetium 99 m Sn colloid, or a combination. Detection can occur via direct visualization or using a γ probe. Based on the data from many individual studies using a combination of these techniques, an average of 1.5 to 4.1 sentinel lymph nodes were detected with sensitivity ranging from 72.7% to 93%, specificity of 75%, accuracy of 74% to 100%, and negative predictive value of 50%.[41,71–76] Limitations of SLNbx include a high false-negative rate in tumors that cause lymphatic obstruction resulting in tracer flowing to secondary negative nodes, skip metastasis, and surgeon experience.[41,77,78]

During the 2009 American Society of Clinical Oncology (ASCO) meeting, The Japan Society of Sentinel Node Navigation Surgery study group reported their findings from a multicenter prospective trial for sentinel node mapping by dual tracer (combined isosulfan blue dye and technetium 99 m tin colloid) injection. They found that 397 patients with early gastric cancer (clinical T1N0M0 or T2N0M0 with primary lesion <4 cm) underwent lymph node mapping. Detection rate was 97.5% (387/397), average number of nodes sampled was 5.6, with a sensitivity of 93%, accuracy of 99% (383/387), and false-negative rate of 7.0%.[79] Based on these data, SLNbx was found to be feasible. Although it may be of limited use in patients with advanced disease, those with early gastric cancer (clinically N0) could potentially benefit from a limited nodal dissection if SLNbx is negative, thereby improving their quality of life.[41,74,80] Furthermore, laparoscopic gastrectomy without formal lymphadenectomy would be easier to perform in those patients who tested SLN-negative.

GASTRIC RESECTION

Surgical resection is the only curative option for gastric cancer. The primary goal of surgery is to remove all gross and microscopic tumors.[81,82] The stomach is a well-vascularized organ with an extensive submucosal lymphatic network, which promotes lymphatic spread of disease. Compared with intestinal type, DGCA has a more aggressive pattern of submucosal spread, and a larger resection margin of 5 cm (vs 3 cm for intestinal type) is recommended.[83] Intraoperative frozen section margin analysis is an important component of operative management to limit the positive margin rate. The extent of gastric resection, whether total gastrectomy (TG) or subtotal gastrectomy (SG) should be performed, has been assessed through several prospective studies. A limited resection can provide disease clearance but minimize patient morbidity. The data are summarized in **Table 4**.[84–86] In all 3 studies, TG was associated with higher morbidity, and did not provide a survival advantage.

Quality of life (QOL) is another important factor in comparing operative procedures. Davies and colleagues[87] compared the QOL of patients with distal gastric cancers undergoing either a TG or SG as measured by 5 questionnaires to measure functional outcome (the Rotterdam Symptom Checklist, the Troidl Index, the Hospital Anxiety and Depression Scale, Activities of Daily Living score, and Visick grade). They found that there were no differences in QOL between the groups before the operation. However, at the 1-year mark and immediately after operation, the SG group had significantly better QOL than the TG group.[87]

Surgery for Proximal Gastric Cancer

Gastric cancers that arise within the proximal portion of the stomach may carry worse prognosis than those that are more distal.[88,89] The question arises whether TG or proximal subtotal gastrectomy (PSG) is better for proximal gastric cancers. Although no randomized controlled trials exist examining this question, Harrison and colleagues[90] conducted a large retrospective study of 391 patients to determine whether the type of operation (TG vs PSG) for proximal gastric cancer affects outcome. They excluded patients who underwent esophagogastrectomy and found

Table 4
Prospective randomized trials addressing extent of gastric resection

Author	Stages	Resection (n)	5-y Survival (%)	Morbidity n (%)	Mortality n (%)	Comments
Gouzi et al,[84] 1989	I–III	SG (93) TG (76)	48 48	32 (34) 25 (32)	3 (3) 1 (1)	Multicenter
Robertson et al,[85] 1994	I–IV	SG (25) TG (30)	45[a] 35	0[a] 24	0 (0) 1 (3)	Single center SG included D1 TG included D3
Bozzetti et al,[86] 1999	I–IV	SG (315) TG (303)	65.3 62.4	N/A —	N/A —	Multicenter

Abbreviation: NA, data not available.
[a] *P* = .05.

that there was no significant difference in the 5-year survival between the 2 groups (43% for PSG and 41 for TG). These findings suggest that PSG with adequate negative margins is oncologically acceptable for select patients. However, recovery from a proximal gastric resection with esophagogastrectomy is often less straightforward secondary to bile reflux esophagitis; thus, despite the defined oncologic soundness of proximal gastrectomy, the authors are not in favor of its use.

RECONSTRUCTION FOLLOWING TG

There are numerous reconstructive options that exist after TG and there is no consensus as to the best procedure, indicating that none are entirely satisfactory.[91] The most common option is the end-to-side esophagojejunostomy with distal drainage of the duodenum by Roux-en-Y enteroenterostomy.[91] Several investigators have assessed the role of jejunal (J) pouch reconstruction to aid in postoperative recovery.

A prospective study by Kurita and colleagues[92] randomized 30 patients who underwent TG to a Roux-en-Y reconstruction either with or without a J-pouch. They found that there was no difference between the 2 groups in dietary intake, body weight, or abdominal complaints. One J-pouch had to be resected because of poor emptying. They concluded that there was no advantage of J-pouch reconstruction following TG.

Gertler and colleagues[91] conducted a meta-analysis assessing the value of pouch formation as a gastric substitute after TG. They reviewed data from 13 randomized control trials; 9 comparing Roux-en-Y reconstructions with and without pouch and 4 comparing jejunal interpositions with and without pouch. The results indicate that creation of a pouch can be done safely without increased morbidity or mortality and without significantly increasing the operative time or length of hospital stay. QOL, as measured by the Gastrointestinal Quality of Life Index, was also found to be significantly better in patients with pouch reconstruction compared with those without regarding postgastrectomy symptoms, eating capability, and body weight.[93] This difference even increased with time from 6 to 12 and 24 months after surgery. In addition, on meta-analysis, pouch reconstruction after TG was determined to be beneficial for patients undergoing curative resection (R0) with expected long-term survival as opposed to palliative resection.[91] Caution needs to be taken in interpreting the data because many studies had small sample sizes and reconstructive techniques were heterogeneous.

The authors generally favor Roux-en-Y esophagojejunal reconstruction without pouch formation because of its simplicity. Pouch reconstruction is used selectively in younger patients who express interest in this method.

EXTENDED LYMPHADENECTOMY

One of the most controversial areas in gastric cancer management is the appropriate extent of nodal dissection. Lymph node involvement is one of the most important independent prognostic factors in gastric cancer. Although, to date, no randomized trial has shown a survival benefit for patients having a more extended node dissection, it is generally agreed that pathologic evaluation of higher lymph node counts provides more accurate staging. The degree of lymph node dissection was traditionally based on the Japanese staging system in which nodal stations were assigned into groups N1, N2, or N3. If a dissection removes N1 nodes (perigastric nodes along the left and right pericardial nodes, lesser and greater curvature, suprapyloric and infrapyloric), it is classified as a D1 dissection. Anything less than a D1 is considered D0 dissection. D2 dissection is D1 plus removal of nodes along the left gastric artery, common hepatic artery, celiac trunk, and splenic artery. D3 is a D2 plus removal of nodes along the hepatoduodenal ligament and root of the mesentery. A D4 is D3 plus removal of para-aortic and paracolic lymph nodes. A D1 dissection is classified as conservative lymph node dissection (CLND) and D2 to D4 dissections are considered extended lymph node dissections (ELND).

In Japan, numerous retrospective and observational studies show improved survival for patients undergoing ELND compared with CLND. Kodama and colleagues[94] found a significant 5-year survival benefit in 454 patients undergoing a D2 or D3 dissection compared with the 254 patients undergoing a D0 or D1 dissection (39% vs 18%, $P<.001$). Likewise, Maruyama and colleagues[95] found improved 5-year survival in D2 lymphadenectomy versus D1 in a study with 6537 patients (63.8% vs 41.2%). Based on these and similar findings from other retrospective studies, ELND is more commonly practiced in the East compared with the West.

Results from prospective trials do not corroborate those from the retrospective studies mentioned earlier. Summary data from the prospective trails can be found in **Table 5**. The Dutch Gastric Cancer Group conducted one of the largest randomized prospective trials.[96] In the study, 711 patients from 80 centers were randomized to undergo gastrectomy with a D1 or D2 dissection. All stages of disease (I–IV) were included and they found that the D2 group had higher morbidity (43% vs 25%, $P<.001$) and mortality (10% vs 4%, $P = .004$) than the D1 group.[96] After a median follow-up of 72 months, no survival advantage was seen in the ELND group. The investigators concluded that routine D2 dissection could not be supported in patients with gastric cancer. Several limitations of the trial were that greater than 50% of specimens in the D2 group lacked at least 2 of the lymph node stations required for completion of the procedure, and 42% of D1 specimens had too many nodal stations included (contamination).

The next prospective study was conducted by the Medical Research Council (MRC) in the United Kingdom. In the trial, 400 patients were randomized to gastrectomy with

Table 5
Summary of prospective randomized trials addressing extent of lymphadenectomy

Author	Stages	LND (n)	5-y survival (%)	Morbidity n (%)	Mortality n (%)
Dent et al,[99] 1988	I–IIIA	D1 (22)	78 (3-y)	3 (4)	0 (0)
		D2 (21)	76 (3-y)	7 (9)	0 (0)
Robertson et al,[85] 1994	I–IV	D1 (25)	45	0 (0)	0 (0)
		D3 (30)	35	24 (57)[a]	1 (3)
Bonenkamp et al,[109] (Dutch trial) 1995	I–IV	D1 (380)	45	94 (25)	15 (4)
		D2 (331)	47	142 (43)[a]	32 (10)[a]
Cushieri et al,[97,110] (UK MRC trial) 1996 and 1999	I–IIIB	D1 (200)	35	55 (28)	13 (7)
		D2 (200)	33	92 (46)[a]	26 (13)[a]
Degiuli et al,[98] (IGCSG trial) 2004	I–IIB	D1 (76)	—	8 (11)	1 (1.3)
		D2 (86)	—	14 (16)	0 (0)
Wu et al,[100,101] (Taiwanese trial) 2004, 2006	I-IV	D1 (110)	54	8 (7)	0 (0)
		D3 (111)	60[a]	19 (17)[a]	0 (0)

Abbreviations: IGCSG, Italian Gastric Cancer Study Group; LND, lymph node dissection; MRC, Medical Research Council.

[a] $P<.05$.

either a D1 or D2 dissection. Patients had stages I to IIIB disease and, like the Dutch trial, they found that morbidity and mortality were significantly greater in the D2 than the D1 group (morbidity 46% vs 28%, mortality 13% vs 6.5%).[97] The higher morbidity and mortality in the D2 group was explained, in part, by the concomitant distal pancreatectomy and splenectomy (52% in D2 group, 4% in D1 group).

In a recent prospective series, the Italian Gastric Cancer Study Group (IGCSG) randomized patients to undergo either a D1 or D2 nodal dissection. They similarly found that there were no significant differences in morbidity or mortality between the 2 groups.[98] Long-term survival data were not yet available.

Two other smaller randomized controlled trials were also conducted. Dent and colleagues[99] in South Africa randomized 43 patients to D1 or D2 dissection and found that there was no survival benefit in the ELND group. However, only 11% of patients in the trial were able to be randomized, significantly restricting the power of the study. Nonetheless, no survival benefit was seen.

In another smaller randomized trial, Robertson and colleagues,[85] compared D1plus SG with D3 plus TG in 55 patients with antral cancer. They found that 5-year survival was better in the D1 group than the D3 group (45% vs 35%). Morbidity and mortality were also higher in the ELND group, which was attributed, in part, to complications associated with pancreatectomy and splenectomy.[85]

The only randomized trial supporting ELND was conducted by Wu and colleagues[100,101] in Taiwan. In this single-institution trial, 221 patients were randomized to undergo either a D3 or D1 dissection. The data indicate that morbidity was higher after D3 than after D1 resection (17.1% vs 7.3%, P = .012) but there was no procedure-related mortality in either group. At the 5-year mark, OS was significantly better in the D3 group than in the D1 group (59.5% vs 53.6%, P = .041).[100,101] When this trial was conducted, the classification system of lymph nodes was based on nodal compartments and, therefore, N2 and N3 nodes may have been removed in D1 dissections.[102]

In a recent meta-analysis by the Cochrane Collaboration examining both randomized and nonrandomized trials, there was no significant difference in survival between a D1 and D2 dissection.[103,104] They did find that the data supported D2 dissection in T3 or higher tumors, resulting in a 32% reduction in mortality; however, a small number of patients were used in the analysis.[103] Based on data from the randomized trials, there was increased postoperative mortality in the ELND group, which was attributed to risks associated with pancreatectomy, splenectomy, and surgeon inexperience.[103,104]

In summary, based on the trials mentioned earlier, the retrospective studies suggest improved survival in patients undergoing ELND, but this is not confirmed in prospective studies. With an experienced surgeon, a D2 lymphadenectomy can be performed safely and provides more accurate staging information.

It is our current practice to perform a D2 nodal dissection to ensure adequate staging and minimize patient morbidity.

SPLENECTOMY

The lymphatic drainage of the stomach is intimately related to the spleen, and several reports show that 15% to 27% of patients with gastric cancer have nodal disease in the splenic hilum.[105–108] Splenectomy and distal pancreatectomy are sometimes performed at the time of gastrectomy to thoroughly clear these nodal basins in patients with more proximal gastric cancers. Based on the data in the Dutch and MRC/UK trials, the increased morbidity and mortality seen in ELND was greatly attributed to performance of splenectomy and pancreaticosplenectomy.[109,110]

In a retrospective study, Kasakura and colleagues[111] reviewed 1938 patients who underwent gastrectomy with concomitant splenectomy, pancreaticosplenectomy, or gastrectomy alone. They found that the splenectomy and pancreaticosplenectomy groups had more proximal tumors, advanced T/N stages, and poorer histologic grades. This group also had higher postoperative morbidity comprising pancreatic fistulae (31.4% vs 0.5%, $P<.0001$), anastomotic leaks (15.2% vs 5.0%, $P<.0001$), and intra-abdominal abscesses (18.1% vs 1.0%, $P<.0001$). They also found higher rates of peritoneal (35% vs 29%, $P<.0001$) and local recurrences (14% vs 10%, $P = .0007$) in the splenectomy and pancreaticosplenectomy groups.[111]

In a prospective trial conducted by Yu and colleagues,[112] 207 patients were randomized to undergo TG with or without splenectomy. They found that although there was an association of the splenectomy group with higher morbidity, mortality, higher incidence of positive lymph nodes at the splenic hilum and splenic artery, statistical significance was not reached.

Csendes and colleagues[113] randomized 187 patients to TG and D2 lymphadenectomy either with or without splenectomy. They found that the splenectomy group (n = 90) had higher septic complications than the nonsplenectomy group (n = 97, $P<.04$). The investigators concluded that splenectomy should only be performed in patients with macroscopic disease involving the spleen or perisplenic nodes. In summary, the data do not support prophylactic splenectomy for curative resection.

LAPAROSCOPIC SURGERY

With the advances in surgical technology and surgeon skill, laparoscopic surgery is increasingly moving into the forefront of oncologic surgery. Laparoscopic colectomy for colon cancer is now routine; however, the biology of gastric cancer poses the potential additional risks with laparoscopic gastrectomy of peritoneal seeding and port site recurrence in association with pneumoperitoneum.[59] In the revised Japanese Gastric Cancer Treatment Guidelines, laparoscopy-assisted gastrectomy is classified as an investigational procedure eligible for stage IA and IB cancers only.[114] Many retrospective studies have shown that laparoscopic gastrectomy with D2 lymphadenectomy can be performed safely with less blood loss but with lengthier operative times.[115–118]

A multicenter prospective randomized trial conducted by Kim and colleagues[119] examined the morbidity and mortality of laparoscopic gastrectomy versus open gastrectomy in Korea. Patients underwent either a D1 or D2 lymphadenectomy with Billroth I or II, or Roux-en-Y reconstructions. In an interim report of the data, they found that, in the 342 patients (laparoscopy n = 179; open n = 163), there were no significant differences in postoperative complications (laparoscopy 10.5%, open 14.7%, $P = .137$) or mortality (laparoscopy 1.1%, open 0%, $P = .497$).

In a Western prospective trial, 59 patients were randomized to undergo laparoscopic (n = 30) or open (n = 29) SG for distal gastric cancer. Patients underwent a D1 or D2 lymphadenectomy with either a Roux-en-Y or Billroth II reconstruction. The investigators found no significant differences in the number of lymph nodes retrieved (average of 33.4 in open and 30.0 in laparoscopic group, $P>.05$), operative mortality (open 6.7%, laparoscopy 3.3%, $P>.05$), and 5-year survival (open 55.7%, laparoscopy 58.9%, $P>.05$).[120]

In summary, laparoscopic surgery for gastric cancer can yield similar morbidity, mortality, and number of lymph nodes as open cases in the hands of an experienced surgeon. Although the studies do show promising short-term outcomes, long-term data in a randomized trial are still lacking.

ENDOSCOPIC RESECTION

With advances in technology, endoscopic management of gastric cancer is growing. Endoscopic mucosal resection (EMR) and endoscopic submucosal dissection (ESD) are such advances for local treatment of early lesions. The purpose of these procedures is to allow for the diagnosis and treatment of mucosa-based gastric lesions.[121] EMR uses suction through an endoscope to create a pseudopolyp of the mucosal lesion that can then be removed via a snare.[121] ESD involved submucosal injection of a viscous fluid followed by dissection and excision with a cutting instrument.[121] Comparisons between EMR and ESD are listed in **Table 6**.

According to the Japanese Gastric Cancer Association, guidelines for EMR are:

1. Well-differentiated adenocarcinoma
2. A tumor ≤20 mm in elevated type
3. A tumor ≤10 mm in depressed type
4. Not associated with peptic ulcer
5. Invasion limited to the mucosa.[58,122,123]

The obvious advantages of these approaches are gastric preservation and avoidance of laparotomy or even laparoscopy. However, there are some concerns associated with these endoscopic techniques, such as the possibility of higher local recurrence rates and the failure to perform a staging lymphadenectomy. EMR often results in piecemeal resection of the index lesion, especially for tumors larger than 20 mm. Studies have found that recurrence rates were higher in piecemeal resections, because of incorrect pathologic assessment of the multiple specimens obtained.[124,125]

EMR allows for the depth of the lesion to be determined during the time of the procedure. Retrospective studies have indicated that complete resection was achievable in 73.9% to 97.7%.[126–128] In a prospective study by Ida and colleagues,[124] the complete excision rate for small, intramucosal lesions was 71.9% but 46.3% for large differentiated carcinomas 2.1 to 4 cm in size. In cases in which there was incomplete resection, repeat treatment in select cases did result in complete cure.[124,129] Retrospective studies examining long-term outcomes have found similar 5-year survivals between EMR and surgery.[123,130,131]

ESD was developed to address this concern. ESD allows for en bloc resection, improved histopathologic assessment, and potentially fewer local recurrences.[132,133]

Table 6
Comparison of EMR and ESD

	EMR	ESD
Lesion size	Lesions <1.5 cm	Lesions >1.5 cm
Lesion characteristic	Flat, raised lesions	Flat lesions
Type of resection	Resect mucosal and superficial submucosal lesions	Resect deeper submucosal lesions
Method of resection	Suction-based snare	Dissection knife
Resection specimen removal	Usually in fragments (piecemeal)	Usually en bloc
Complications	Lower	Higher
Recurrence	Higher	Lower

Data from Wang KK, Prasad G, Tian J. Endoscopic mucosal resection and endoscopic submucosal dissection in esophageal and gastric cancers. Curr Opin Gastroenterol 2010;26(5):453–8.

Early feasibility studies in Japan and Asia show promising results and ESD is commonly practiced. In the West, data are limited, there are a limited number of early gastric cancer cases compared with the East, and there is a steep learning curve. A large European retrospective study conducted by Probst and colleagues[134] examined 91 ESDs for early gastric cancer and adenomas. They found that ESD was possible in 93.4% of cases, with a recurrence rate of 5.6% and no mortality. ESD is still in the early stages of development but shows tremendous promise as an alternative to open procedures.

Another issue is that of nodal staging. Patients with early gastric cancer, defined as lesions confined to the mucosa or submucosa, still carry a 10% to 20% risk of lymph node metastases.[135] A study by Soetikno and colleagues[136] examined the risk of lymph node involvement in 5625 early gastric cancer cases to justify expanding criteria for local treatment. Based on their findings, the criteria for EMR were expanded to:

1. Mucosal cancer of the intestinal type irrespective of the size of the lesion when no ulceration is present
2. Mucosal cancer of the intestinal type with a diameter of less than 30 mm when ulceration is present
3. Submucosal invasive cancer of the intestinal type when the diameter is restricted to 30 mm and when submucosal invasion is restricted to less than 500 μm.

In summary, in endemic areas of the world such as Japan and Korea where approximately 50% of patients present with early gastric cancer, procedures such as EMR and ESD are common practice.[129,137,138] However, in the West, where such early presentations are rare and operator experience is minimal, endoscopic procedures should be individualized and limited to specialized centers with multidisciplinary input.

ADVANCED SURGICAL PROCEDURES

Natural Orifice Transluminal Endoscopic Surgery

Natural orifice transluminal endoscopic surgery (NOTES) is considered by many to represent the next evolution in minimally invasive surgery.[139] NOTES in gastric cancer is only beginning to be examined and is typically performed as a hybrid procedure along with laparoscopy. Early feasibility studies conducted for mucosal and submucosal lesions revealed minimal to no adverse postoperative events, acceptable operative times and blood loss, and adequate lymph node harvest.[140,141] NOTES is also being investigated for sentinel lymph node biopsy. A study by Cahill and colleagues[142] proved that lymphatic mapping and node biopsy are achievable in a porcine model; however, human studies are lacking. The ability to reliably close a full-thickness gastrostomy also needs to be perfected before NOTES can move into the mainstream of gastric surgery. Although initial feasibility studies are promising, many technical aspects need to be worked out and outcome studies completed in a prospective manner.

Robot-assisted Surgery

Like NOTES, robot-assisted surgery (RAS) is a product of innovations in surgical technology. Robotic surgery was originally designed to minimize the shortcomings of laparoscopic surgery. RAS provides articulated movement, elimination of the physiologic tremor, and a steady camera platform that allows for more precise instrument movement and dissections.[143] In one of the largest series, Song and colleagues[143] presented their experience in 100 patients with early gastric cancer who underwent robot-assisted gastrectomy using the da Vinci Surgical System. There were 33 patients who underwent TG and 67 patients who had subtotal gastrectomies with

D1 dissections. They found that the average total operation time was 231 minutes, average hospital length of stay was 7.8 days, mean number of lymph nodes recovered was 36.7, and there was no mortality.

Although this was one of many studies examining the safety of robot-assisted gastrectomy, multicenter, prospective, and comparative studies need to be conducted.

CHEMOTHERAPY AND RADIATION FOR RESECTABLE DISEASE

Neoadjuvant Therapy

Chemotherapy

Even after potentially curative surgery, OS at 5 years for patients with gastric adenocarcinoma remains as low as 20% to 30%.[144,145] Theoretically, administration of chemotherapy before surgical resection can address micrometastatic lesions and downstage disease. It also allows for an in vivo assessment of chemotherapeutic efficacy in those patients with measurable disease (primary or perigastric nodal disease) on imaging. Some concerns regarding preoperative therapy are progression of disease before resection and the potential for surgery-preventing toxicity. In reality, the patients who progress on preoperative therapy may be spared unnecessary laparotomy, because their disease is likely beyond surgical therapy at presentation. Toxicity remains an issue, because the platinum-based regimens that are often used can be difficult to tolerate.

A study by Lowy and colleagues[146] found that, in the 83 patients treated with neoadjuvant chemotherapy, responders had a higher 5-year survival than nonresponders (83% vs 31%, $P<.001$), and response to chemotherapy was the strongest predictor of survival. A recent meta-analysis of trials examining preoperative therapy was performed by Li and colleagues[147] (**Table 7**). Twelve studies with 1868 patients were assessed for survival following surgery for locally advanced gastric cancer with either neoadjuvant chemotherapy or surgery alone, with a median follow-up time of 3 years.[148–159] The neoadjuvant group had a marginal improvement in OS compared with the control group (48.1% vs 46.9%, odds ratio [OR] 1.27, 95% CI 1.04–1.55).[147] Three studies found 3-year progression-free survival to be higher in the neoadjuvant compared with the control group (41.1% vs 27.5%, OR 1.85, 95% CI 1.39–2.46).[147–150] A significant downstaging effect was also seen in the neoadjuvant group compared with controls (49.9% vs 37.5%, OR 1.71, 95% CI 1.26–2.33), and complete resection (R0) was found to be higher in the neoadjuvant group (75.2% vs 66.9%, OR 1.51, 95% CI 1.19–1.91).[147,148,150–152,156,158,160] In a subgroup analysis, the investigators determined that patients who had gastric cancer with later stages of disease (pT3-4) benefited more from neoadjuvant therapy than those at earlier stages (pT1–2) when OS rate was the end point and monotherapy was inferior to a multitherapy regimens.[147] Although no conclusions regarding the best chemotherapeutic regimen could be drawn, the analysis did reveal that combination therapy and intravenous administration were more effective than monotherapy, oral administration, or intra-arterial administration.[147]

The role of neoadjuvant therapy for resectable disease was examined in several recent prospective studies. The Dutch Gastric Cancer Group randomized 59 patients to receive surgery alone (n = 30) or 4 courses of chemotherapy (n = 29) using 5-fluorouracil (5-FU), doxorubicin, and methotrexate (FAMTX). The trial was closed early because of poor accrual and, after a median follow-up time of 83 months, they concluded that no survival benefit was seen with this regimen (median survival FAMTX, 18 months; median survival surgery alone, 30 months; $P = .17$).[151] Several criticisms of the study are poor preoperative staging, limited statistical power, and limited efficacy of the FAMTX regimen.[161]

Table 7
Trials examining neoadjuvant chemotherapy in advanced gastric cancer

Author	Country	Patients (n)		Neoadjuvant Group		Control Group		
		Neoadjuvant	Control	Preoperative Therapy	Postoperative Therapy	Preoperative Therapy	Postoperative Therapy	Median Follow-up (mo)
Schuhmacher et al,[148] 2009	Germany	72	72	5-FU + DDP	None	None	None	53
Boige et al,[149] 2007	France	113	111	FP	FP	None	None	68
Cunningham et al,[150] 2006	United Kingdom	250	253	ECF	ECF	None	None	47
Hartgrink et al,[151] 2004	Holland	27	29	FAMTX	None	None	None	83
Nio et al,[152] 2004	Japan	102	193	UFT (oral)	CT	None	CT	83
Zhang et al,[153] 2004	China	37	54	Intravenous (no details)	None	None	None	NR
Kobayashi et al,[154] 2000	Japan	91	80	5-FU (oral)	CT	None	None	NR
Wang et al,[155] 2000	China	30	30	5-FU (oral)	None	None	None	NR
Takiguchi et al,[191] 2000	Japan	123	139	5-FU ± DDP	None	None	None	NR
Lygidakis et al,[156] 1999	Greece	39	19	IP	CT	None	None	NR
Kang et al,[160] 1996	Korea	53	54	PEF	PEF	None	PEF	>36
Masuyama et al,[157] 1994	Japan	24	98	EAP (IA)	None	None	None	>36
Yonemura et al,[158] 1993	Japan	29	26	PMUE	None	None	PMUE	24
Nishioka et al,[159] 1982	Japan	64	59	5-FU (oral)	CT	None	CT	>60

Abbreviations: CT, chemotherapy; DDP, cisplatin; EAP, epirubicin/adriamycin/cisplatin; ECF, epirubicin/cyclophosphamide/5-FU; FAMTX, 5-FU/adriamycin/methotrexate; FP, 5-FU/cisplatin; IP, intraperitoneal; NAC, neoadjuvant chemotherapy; PEF, cisplatin/epirubicin/5-FU; PMUE, cisplatin/mitomycin C/etoposide/UFT; UFT, tegafur/uracil; 5-FU, 5-fluorouracil.

From Li W, Qin J, Sun YH, et al. Neoadjuvant chemotherapy for advanced gastric cancer: a meta-analysis. World J Gastroenterol 2010;16(44):5621–8; with permission.

A pivotal study on the role of chemotherapy for resectable gastric cancer was the Medical Research Council Adjuvant Gastric Cancer Infusional Chemotherapy (MAGIC) trial. Patients with stage II to IVA gastric cancer (74%), distal esophageal (11%), and gastroesophageal junction (15%) cancers were randomized to receive perioperative chemotherapy (n = 250) or surgery alone (n = 253). The chemotherapy regimen consisted of 3 cycles of epirubicin, cisplatin, and 5-FU (ECF) before and after surgery. Data indicated that 5-year survival was better (36% vs 23%, HR 0.75, 95% CI 0.60–0.93, *P* = .009), progression-free survival was longer (HR for progression 0.66, 95% CI 0.53–0.81, *P*<.001), and local recurrence rates were lower (14.4% perioperative chemotherapy group; 20.6% surgery group) in the ECF arm.[150] Tumor downstaging was also seen for both T and N stage. Limitations of the trial include inability to determine the contribution of preoperative versus postoperative chemotherapy on survival because of the trial design, and the differential impact on distal esophageal and gastroesophageal junction tumors could not be assessed because they were both included in the study.[161]

Ongoing studies include the MAGIC-B trial conducted by The UK National Cancer Research Institute Upper Gastrointestinal Clinical Studies Group. They are evaluating the addition of bevacizumab to perioperative epirubicin, cisplatin, and capecitabine (ECX). Approximately 1100 patients with resectable distal esophageal, gastroesophageal junction, and gastric adenocarcinoma will be enrolled. In another trial, the Dutch Gastric Cancer Group will evaluate 788 patients with resectable gastric cancer receiving preoperative and postoperative ECX followed by concurrent chemoradiation with cisplatin and capecitabine after resection (see **Table 7**).

Radiotherapy

Radiotherapy in the neoadjuvant setting offers several advantages such as increased target accuracy and efficacy before the tumor bed and vascular supply is disrupted by surgical intervention.[161] In a large prospective study in China, investigators randomized 370 patients with locally advanced gastric cancer of the cardia to preoperative radiation (40 Gy) or surgery alone.[162] The 5-year survival was significantly higher in the radiation group than in the surgery-alone group (30.1% vs 19.8%, *P* = .009). In addition, a lower recurrence rate (39% vs 52%, *P* = .025) and increased resectability (90% vs 79%, *P* = .01) were seen in the radiation group.[162]

In a European study, Skoropad and colleagues[163] randomized 102 patients to either preoperative radiation or surgery alone. In a 20-year follow-up period, no significant improvement in survival was seen. Patients in this study underwent exploratory laparotomy before enrollment to ensure absence of peritoneal disease. Currently no randomized trials support the administration of neoadjuvant radiotherapy rather than surgery alone.

Chemoradiotherapy

The local control benefits of concomitant neoadjuvant chemotherapy and radiotherapy in cancers of the rectum and esophagus are established.[164–167] Several groups have examined the use of chemoradiation for gastric cancer. A phase II clinical trial conducted by Ajani and colleagues[168] evaluated the efficacy of cisplatin, 5-FU, and leucovorin, followed by concurrent chemoradiation using infusional 5-FU, before surgery. They found a pathologic complete response in 30% of patients and partial response in 24%. There was significant downstaging of tumors and patients who achieved complete or partial response lived longer than nonresponders (63.9 vs 12.6 months, *P* = .03).[168]

The Radiation Therapy Oncology Group trial 99-04 similarly examined chemoradiation therapy in patients with resectable gastric cancer. The regimen included induction cisplatin, infusional 5-FU, and leucovorin for 2 cycles, followed by concurrent chemoradiation with infusional 5-FU plus weekly paclitaxel before surgery.[169] Of the 43 patients (49 originally enrolled), a pathologic complete response was seen in 26% and R0 resection completed in 77%.[168]

Although many of the studies show promising results, large prospective randomized trials are lacking. Based on these studies, neoadjuvant therapy can be administered in carefully selected patients, with radiotherapy alone having limited benefit.

Adjuvant Therapy

Chemotherapy

Many trials have evaluated the efficacy of adjuvant chemotherapy alone for resected gastric cancer, but results of this approach have not been impressive.[161,170–172] Because these trials suffer from low power, several meta-analyses were performed to combine reports and address this deficiency in study design (**Table 8**).[161] Overall, a modest improvement in OS was seen for patients receiving adjuvant chemotherapy; however, because of the heterogeneity of the studies, determination of the best regimen or target patient population could not be defined. As examples, one meta-analysis showed benefit of adjuvant chemotherapy for Asian patients, whereas another for lymph node–positive patients (**Table 9** summarizes results from select trials for adjuvant therapy).[173,174]

Table 8
Meta-analysis of randomized controlled trials of adjuvant chemotherapy in gastric cancer

Author	Number of Studies	Number of Patients	OR for Death/HR for Mortality	Features of Analysis
Hermans et al,[215] 1993	11	2096	OR = 0.88 (95 % CI 0.78–1.08)	Adjuvant chemotherapy, immunotherapy, intraperitoneal therapy, and radiotherapy trials
Earle et al,[173] 1999	13	1990	OR = 0.80 (95% CI 0.66–0.97)	Adjuvant systemic chemotherapy trials only Exclusion of Asian studies
Mari et al,[216] 2000	21	3658	HR = 0.82 (95% CI 0.75–0.89)	Adjuvant systemic chemotherapy trials only Use of HRs to account for time of event
Panzini et al,[217] 2002	17	3118	OR = 0.72 (95% CI 0.62–0.84)	Adjuvant systemic chemotherapy trials only Exclusion of trials with incompletely resected patients
Janunger et al,[174] 2002	21	3962	Overall: HR = 0.84 (95% CI 0.74–0.96) Western studies: HR = 0.96 (95% CI 0.83–1.12) Asian Studies: HR = 0.58 (95% CI 0.44–0.76)	Adjuvant systemic chemotherapy trials only Neoadjuvant chemotherapy and intraperitoneal chemotherapy trials included in descriptive analysis Separate analysis of Asian (n = 4) and Western (n = 17) adjuvant systemic chemotherapy studies showed benefit in Asian only

From Ng K, Meyerhardt JA, Fuchs CS. Adjuvant and neoadjuvant approaches in gastric cancer. Cancer J 2007;13(3):168–74; with permission.

Table 9
Selected randomized control trials of adjuvant therapies in gastric cancer

Author	Treatment	N	Stage	Survival (%)	*P*-value
Gastrointestinal Study Group,[192] 1982	Surgery alone	82	N/A	32[a]	NS
	Semustine Fluorouracil Surgery	93		46[a]	
Higgins et al,[193] 1983	Surgery alone	66	T1–4, NX, M0	38[d]	NS
	Semustine, 5-FU Surgery	68		39[d]	
Engstrom et al,[194] 1985	Surgery alone	89	T1–4, NX, M0	32.7[c]	NS
	Semustine Fluorouracil Fluorouracil Surgery	91		36.6[c]	
Italian Gastrointestinal Study Group[195] 1988	Surgery alone	69	N/A	29	NS
	Semustine, 5-FU Surgery	75		28	
	Semustine, 5-FU, Levamisole Surgery	69		30	
Coombes et al,[196] 1990	Surgery alone	148	II–III	35	NS
	Fluorouracil Doxorubicin Mitomycin C Surgery	133		46	
Estape et al,[197] 1991	Surgery alone	148	I–III	48[a]	<0.01
	5-FU Doxorubicin Mitomycin C Surgery	133		84[a]	
Krook et al,[198] 1991	Surgery alone	64	I–IV	33[a]	NS
	Fluorouracil Doxorubicin Surgery	63		32[a]	
Kim et al,[199] 1992	Surgery alone	94	III	24.4	<0.05
	5-FU, surgery, mitomycin C	77		29.8	
	5-FU, surgery, mitomycin C Picibanil	159		45.3	
Grau et al,[200] 1993	Surgery alone	66	I–III	26[a]	<0.025
	Mitomycin C Surgery	68		41[a]	
Hallissey et al,[176] 1994	Surgery alone	145	II–IV	20[a]	NS
	5-FU, surgery Doxorubicin Mitomycin C	138		19[a]	
	Radiotherapy, surgery	153		12[a]	

(*continued on next page*)

Table 9
(continued)

Author	Treatment	N	Stage	Survival (%)	*P*-value
Lise et al,[201] 1995	Surgery alone Fluorouracil Doxorubicin Mitomycin C Surgery	159 155	II–III	40[a] 43[a]	NS
Macdonald et al,[202] 1995	Surgery alone Fluorouracil Doxorubicin Mitomycin C Surgery	112 109	I–III	32[a] 37[a]	NS
Neri et al,[203] 1996	Surgery alone Epirubicin, 5-FU Folinic acid	48 55	T1–2, N1-2	13[c] 25[c]	<0.01
Nakajima et al,[204] 1999	Surgery alone Mitomycin C Fluorouracil Uracil+tegafur Surgery	288 288	Serosa negative	83[a] 86[a]	NS
Bajetta et al,[205] 2001	Surgery alone Etoposide Fluorouracil Doxorubicin Cisplatin Surgery Leucovorin	136 135	I–IV	48[a] 52[a]	NS
MacDonald et al,[177] 2001	Surgery alone 5-FU, surgery Leucovorin Radiotherapy	275 281	IB–IV M0	27[b] 36[b]	0.005
Nashimoto et al,[206] 2003	Surgery alone Mitomycin C Fluorouracil Cytosine arabinoside Surgery	124 128	I–II	86[a] 91[a]	NS
Popiela et al,[207] 2004	Surgery alone Fluorouracil Doxorubicin Mitomycin C Surgery	52 53	III–IV	27[b] 28[b]	NS
Bouché et al,[208] 2005	Surgery alone Fluorouracil Cisplatin Surgery	140 138	I–IV	42[a] 47[a]	NS
Nitti et al,[209] 2006	Surgery alone Fluorouracil Doxorubicin Leucovorin Methotrexate Surgery	103 103	I–IV	44 43	NS

(*continued on next page*)

Table 9
(*continued*)

Author	Treatment	N	Stage	Survival (%)	*P*-value
Nakajima et al,[210] 2007	Surgery alone Uracil+tegafur Surgery	95 95	II–III	73[a] 86[a]	0.017
Sakuramoto et al,[175] 2007	Surgery alone S-1 Surgery	530 529	II–III	70.1[c] 80.1[c]	0.003
De Vita et al,[211] 2007	Surgery alone Epirubicin Fluorouracil Etoposide Leucovorin Surgery	113 112	I–III	43.5[a] 48[a]	NS
Cascinu et al,[212] 2007	Fluorouracil Leucovorin Surgery Epidoxorubicin Fluorouracil Leucovorin Cisplatin Surgery	196 201	II–III	50[a] 52[a]	NS
Di Costanzo et al,[213] 2008	Surgery alone Cisplatin Epirubicin Fluorouracil Leucovorin Surgery	128 130	IB–IV	48.7[a] 47.6[a]	NS
Kulig et al,[214] 2010	Surgery alone Etoposide Adriamycin Cisplatin Surgery	154 141	I–III	40[a] 44[a]	NS

[a] 5-year survival.
[b] Median survival in months.
[c] 3-year survival.
[d] 3.5-year survival.

A Japanese trial by Sakuramoto and colleagues[175] randomized 1059 patients to surgery alone (n = 530) with greater than or equal to D2 dissection or surgery with adjuvant S-1, an oral fluoropyrimidine (n = 529). The trial was stopped at 1 year after the first interim analysis because of significantly better survival in patients treated with adjuvant S-1. Follow-up data showed that 5-year OS was 70.1% in the surgery arm and 80.1% in the S-1 arm (*P* = .003).

The UK MAGIC trial (mentioned previously) showed improved 5-year survival, progression-free survival, and reduced local recurrence in the ECF arm. Because of the trial design, the contribution of postoperative chemotherapy on survival could not be determined.[150]

The current data support adjuvant chemotherapy despite the modestly positive results from meta-analyses. Given that most trials were conducted in Europe and

Asia, future studies need to validate the survival benefit of adjuvant chemotherapy in a Western patient population.

Radiation

The presence of locoregional recurrence after resection makes radiotherapy an attractive option for gastric cancer. However, gastric cancer is notoriously radioresistant.[161] A prospective randomized trial was conducted by the British Stomach Cancer Group to assess external beam radiation therapy.[176] Four-hundred and thirty-six patients with stage II and III disease who underwent resection were randomized to no therapy, adjuvant radiotherapy, or adjuvant chemotherapy with mitomycin, doxorubicin, and fluorouracil. They found that there was no significant difference in 5-year survival between the groups (20% surgery alone, 12% surgery plus radiotherapy, and 19% surgery plus chemotherapy).[176] Thus far, the benefit of adjuvant radiotherapy alone has not been validated.

Chemoradiotherapy

Although the administration of adjuvant radiotherapy alone for gastric cancer has not been proven, concomitant chemotherapy with radiotherapy does provide a survival benefit for some patients. The US Southwest Oncology Group Intergroup trial (SWOG 9008/INT-0116) by Macdonald and colleagues[177] randomized 556 patients who underwent complete resection for stage IB to IVA gastric or gastroesophageal junction cancer to surgery alone ($n = 275$) or surgery with postoperative chemoradiotherapy ($n = 281$). The regimen consisted of 425 mg/m^2 of 5-FU with leucovorin 20 mg/m^2/d for 5 days followed by 45 Gy of radiation at 180 cGy per day for 5 weeks with modified doses of 5-FU/leucovorin. One month after completion of the radiotherapy, 2 additional 5-day cycles of 5-FU/leucovorin were administered. The initial results of the study were published in 2001 and updated in 2004 with median follow-up of more than 6 years. They found that the surgery plus adjuvant chemoradiotherapy resulted in improved OS (35 vs 26 months, $P = .006$) and disease-free survival (30 vs 19 months, $P<.001$) compared with surgery only.[177,178] One of the strongest criticisms of the study concerned the inadequate extent of lymph node dissection. A D2 nodal dissection was accomplished in 10% of patients and 54% underwent less than a D1 lymphadenectomy. In a subgroup analysis of the patients who underwent D2 dissection, the improvement in overall and disease-free survival was not seen.[171] In addition, the efficacy of bolus 5-FU used in the trial is of question because an analysis of relapse rates showed that 5-FU administration did not have an effect on extra-abdominal relapse (12% with surgery only, 14% with 5-FU). Despite the criticisms, the administration of adjuvant chemoradiotherapy has doubled since the release of the Intergroup INT-0116 trial and can be considered standard of care for patients with stage IB or higher gastric adenocarcinoma.[179,180]

The Cancer and Leukemia Group B (CALGB) 80101 study was developed to assess which chemotherapeutic agent is superior in combination with radiotherapy in the adjuvant setting. This ongoing phase III trial will randomize patients who have undergone curative resection of gastric or gastroesophageal junction cancer to receive either 5-FU or ECF before and after concurrent infusional 5-FU/radiation.

Intraperitoneal therapy

Peritoneal carcinomatosis is common in gastric cancer and is responsible for about 60% of all deaths from this disease.[181] Although systemic chemotherapy is the treatment of choice for disseminated disease, the blood-peritoneal barrier (BPB) prevents these agents from achieving their maximal cytotoxic effect. The BPB is approximately 90 μm in width and consists of a monolayer of mesothelial cells, basement membrane, and submesothelial connective tissue between the basement membrane and capillaries.[181] Studies have shown that, after the intravenous administration of 5-FU, the intraperitoneal concentration of drug is not sufficient to have a cytotoxic effect.[182] Intraperitoneal chemotherapy (IPC) provides the option of administering significantly higher doses of chemotherapeutic agents to the peritoneal surface while avoiding systemic toxicity. Surgery for peritoneal carcinomatosis was once considered futile, but experience in colorectal and appendiceal cancer has justified the use of cytoreductive surgery (CRS).[183] Studies in gastric cancer failed to reveal a survival benefit of CRS alone; however, the combination of IPC and CRS has improved survival.[184–186]

A recent meta-analysis conducted by Yan and colleagues[187] examined the effectiveness and safety of adjuvant IPC for patients with locally advanced resectable gastric cancer. Thirteen randomized control trials were evaluated and 10 included in the meta-analysis that used hyperthermic intraoperative intraperitoneal chemotherapy (HIIC), normothermic intraoperative intraperitoneal chemotherapy (NIIC), early postoperative intraperitoneal chemotherapy (EPIC), delayed postoperative intraperitoneal chemotherapy (DPIC), and combined forms of intraperitoneal chemotherapy. Chemotherapy agents used include mitomycin C, cisplatin (CDDP), and tegafur/uracil (UFT). There was a significant survival benefit with HIIC (HR 0.60, 95% CI 0.43–0.83, $P = .002$) and HIIC combined with EPIC (HR 0.45, 95% CI 0.29–0.68, $P = .0002$).[187] No survival benefit was seen with NIIC, DPIC, or EPIC alone. In addition, downsides of IPC include higher risks of intra-abdominal abscess formation (relative risk [RR] 2.37, 95% CI 1.32–4.26, $P = .003$) and neutropenia (RR 4.33, 95% CI 1.49–12.61, $P = .007$). Although HIIC was shown to improve OS, no conclusions could be drawn about its effect on preventing locoregional recurrence.

At the author's institution, HIIC with CRS is not yet used for patients with peritoneal carcinomatosis from gastric adenocarcinoma.

In summary, perioperative chemotherapy or adjuvant chemoradiotherapy are now considered standard of care for gastric cancer. Therapies such as IPC have not gained acceptance for gastric cancer at this time.

Palliative Gastrectomy for Patients with Stage IV Disease

The aggressive biologic behavior of gastric adenocarcinoma is associated with many patients showing advanced incurable disease at the time of diagnosis. Patients with stage IV malignancy are often marginal surgical candidates for severe operations such as gastrectomy. Several institutions have reported enhanced survival for patients who are diagnosed with stage IV disease and undergo gastrectomy with or without chemotherapy compared with patients treated nonoperatively.[188–191] These retrospective studies suffer from the extreme limitations associated with selection bias of offering surgery for the patients with the best performance status and relegating to nonoperative management patients who are most symptomatic and preterminal. For patients who have stage IV gastric cancer with symptomatic advanced disease, simple gastric decompression can palliate obstructive symptoms, and the anemia associated with advanced gastric cancer rarely benefits from surgical resection. In the author's opinion, palliative gastrectomy should be limited to a small, highly selective subgroup of patients who require palliation to achieve an adequate performance status that would allow treatment with systemic chemotherapy.

SUMMARY

Gastric adenocarcinoma is an aggressive epithelial malignancy responsible for significant cancer-related mortality worldwide. Although many patients in Japan and other

Asian nations present with early stages of the disease, the same is not true for the United States and Europe. As a result, significant differences exist in the screening, surgical treatment, and medical treatment of these patients. Care must be taken in interpreting data to ensure that findings are applicable to a given patient population.

For surgical treatment, resection is based on the location of the malignancy. Small distal tumors are often treated with subtotal gastrectomies, whereas most other lesions require a TG. Concomitant splenectomy or pancreatectomy can substantially add to patient morbidity and potentially mortality and is not recommended unless there is direct organ invasion. With both operative procedures, a negative resection margin confirmed with intraoperative frozen pathology is imperative. Despite the great controversy surrounding the extent of nodal dissection, a D2 dissection can be done as safely as a D1 dissection by an experienced surgeon and provide sufficient lymph nodes for staging.

Data from many retrospective and prospective trials have guided our treatment of gastric cancer. Although there is no consensus on the perfect treatment regimen (chemotherapy alone vs chemoradiotherapy) or drug combination, many agents and modalities exist, allowing for individualized care based on patient morbidities and stage of disease. Neoadjuvant or adjuvant radiotherapy alone has not been validated, whereas chemotherapy or chemoradiotherapy may be used in carefully selected patients. Treatment options for metastatic disease beyond traditional systemic chemotherapy, such as IPC and CRS, are currently being investigated. Regardless of treatment modality, a multidisciplinary team approach is always recommended because it can offer invaluable information and maximal options for the patient. The future of gastric cancer care is promising as advances in technology and knowledge of molecular pathways give rise to new, effective, and innovative treatment options.

REFERENCES

1. Parkin DM, Bray F, Ferlay J, et al. Global cancer statistics, 2002. CA Cancer J Clin 2005;55(2):74–108.
2. Jemal A, Siegel R, Xu J, et al. Cancer statistics, 2010. CA Cancer J Clin 2010; 60(5):277–300.
3. Altekruse SF, Kosary CL, Krapcho M, et al, editors. Surveillance, Epidemiology, and End Results (SEER) Cancer Statistics Review, 1975-2007. National Cancer Institute; 2010. Available at: http://seer.cancer.gov/statfacts/html/stomach.html. Accessed December 28, 2010.
4. Lauren P. The two histological main types of gastric carcinoma: diffuse and so-called intestinal type carcinoma. Acta Pathol Microbiol Scand 1965;64: 31–49.
5. Bollschweiler E, Boettcher K, Hoelscher AH, et al. Is the prognosis for Japanese and German patients with gastric cancer really different? Cancer 1993;71(10): 2918–25.
6. Correa P, Piazuelo MB, Carmargo MC. Etiopathogenesis of gastric cancer. Scand J Surg 2006;95:218–24.
7. Correa P. Human gastric carcinogenesis: a multistep and multifactorial process-First American Cancer Society Award Lecture on Cancer Epidemiology and Prevention. Cancer Res 1992;52:6735–40.
8. Gastric cancer treatment (PDQ) 2010. Available at: http://www.cancer.gov/cancertopics/pdq/treatment/gastric/. Accessed December 28, 2010.
9. Vauhkonen M, Vauhkonen H, Sipponen P. Pathology and molecular biology of gastric cancer. Best Pract Res Clin Gastroenterol 2006;20(4):651–74.

10. Munson JL, O'Mahony R. Radical gastrectomy for cancer of the stomach. Surg Clin North Am 2005;85(5):1021–32, vii.
11. Foschi R, Lucenteforte E, Bosetti C, et al. Family history of cancer and stomach cancer risk. Int J Cancer 2008;123(6):1429–32.
12. Varley JM, McGown G, Thorncroft M, et al. Germ-line mutations of TP53 in Li-Fraumeni families: an extended study of 39 families. Cancer Res 1997; 57(15):3245–52.
13. Vasen HF, Wunen JT, Menko FH, et al. Cancer risk in families with hereditary nonpolyposis colorectal cancer diagnosed by mutation analysis. Gastroenterology 1996;110:1020–7.
14. Fitzgerald RC, Hardwick R, Huntsman D, et al. Hereditary diffuse gastric cancer: updated consensus guidelines for clinical management and directions for future research. J Med Genet 2010;47(7):436–44.
15. Carneiro F, Oliveira C, Seruca R. Pathology and genetics of familial gastric cancer. Int J Surg Pathol 2010;18(Suppl 3):33S–6S.
16. Guilford P, Hopkins J, Harraway J, et al. E-cadherin germline mutations in familial gastric cancer. Nature 1998;392(6674):402–5.
17. Caldas C, Carneiro F, Lynch H, et al. Familial gastric cancer: overview and guidelines for management. J Med Genet 1999;36(12):873–80.
18. Blair V, Martin I, Shaw D, et al. Hereditary diffuse gastric cancer: diagnosis and management. Clin Gastroenterol Hepatol 2006;4(3):262–75.
19. Yao J, Schnirer I, Reddy S, et al. Effects of sex and racial/ethnic group on the pattern of gastric cancer localization. Gastric Cancer 2002;5:208–12.
20. Yeh J, Munn S, Plunkett T, et al. Coexistence of acanthosis nigricans and the sign of Leser-Trelat in a patient with gastric adenocarcinoma: a case report and literature review. J Am Acad Dermatol 2000;42(2):357–62.
21. Maehara Y, Moriguchi S, Kakeji Y, et al. Pertinent risk factors and gastric carcinoma with synchronous peritoneal dissemination or liver metastasis. Surgery 1991;110(5):820–3.
22. Esaki Y, Hirayama R, Hirokawa K. A comparison of patterns of metastasis in gastric cancer by histologic type and age. Cancer 1990;65(9):2086–90.
23. Jemal A, Center MM, DeSantis C, et al. Global patterns of cancer incidence and mortality rates and trends. Cancer Epidemiol Biomarkers Prev 2010;19(8):1893–907.
24. Everett SM, Axon AT. Early gastric cancer in Europe. Gut 1997;41(2):142–50.
25. Maruyama K, Kaminishi M, Hayashi K, et al. Gastric cancer treated in 1991 in Japan: data analysis of nationwide registry. Gastric Cancer 2006;9(2):51–66.
26. Ahn HS, Lee HJ, Yoo MW, et al. Changes in clinicopathological features and survival after gastrectomy for gastric cancer over a 20-year period. Br J Surg 2011;98(2):255–60.
27. Botterweck AA, Schouten LJ, Volovics A, et al. Trends in incidence of adenocarcinoma of the oesophagus and gastric cardia in ten European countries. Int J Epidemiol 2000;29(4):645–54.
28. Devesa SS, Blot WJ, Fraumeni JF Jr. Changing patterns in the incidence of esophageal and gastric carcinoma in the United States. Cancer 1998;83(10): 2049–53.
29. El-Serag H. Time trends of gastroesophageal reflux disease: a systematic review. Clin Gastroenterol Hepatol 2007;5(1):17–26.
30. Mihmanli M, Dilege E, Demir U, et al. The use of tumor markers as predictors of prognosis in gastric cancer. Hepatogastroenterology 2004;51(59):1544–7.
31. Lukaszewicz-Zając M, Mroczko B, Gryko M, et al. Comparison between clinical significance of serum proinflammatory proteins (IL-6 and CRP) and classic

tumor markers (CEA and CA 19-9) in gastric cancer. Clin Exp Med 2011;11(2): 89–96.
32. Dilege E, Mihmanli M, Demir U, et al. Prognostic value of preoperative CEA and CA 19-9 levels in resectable gastric cancer. Hepatogastroenterology 2010; 57(99–100):674–7.
33. Emara M, Cheung P, Grabowski K, et al. Serum levels of matrix metalloproteinase-2 and -9 and conventional tumor markers (CEA and CA 19-9) in patients with colorectal and gastric cancers. Clin Chem Lab Med 2009;47(8):993–1000.
34. Liu X, Cheng Y, Sheng W, et al. Clinicopathologic features and prognostic factors in alpha-fetoprotein-producing gastric cancers: analysis of 104 cases. J Surg Oncol 2010;102(3):249–55.
35. Tsubono Y, Hisamichi S. Screening for gastric cancer in Japan. Gastric Cancer 2000;4(3):9–18.
36. Dooley CP, Larson AW, Stace NH, et al. Double-contrast barium meal and upper gastrointestinal endoscopy. A comparative study. Ann Intern Med 1984;101(4): 538–45.
37. Suzuki H, Gotoda T, Sasako M, et al. Detection of early gastric cancer: misunderstanding the role of mass screening. Gastric Cancer 2006;9(4):315–9.
38. Bhandari S, Shim CS, Kim JH, et al. Usefulness of three-dimensional, multidetector row CT (virtual gastroscopy and multiplanar reconstruction) in the evaluation of gastric cancer: a comparison with conventional endoscopy, EUS, and histopathology. Gastrointest Endosc 2004;59(6):619–26.
39. Chen J, Cheong JH, Yun MJ, et al. Improvement in preoperative staging of gastric adenocarcinoma with positron emission tomography. Cancer 2005; 103(11):2383–90.
40. Kim SK, Kang KW, Lee JS, et al. Assessment of lymph node metastases using 18F-FDG PET in patients with advanced gastric cancer. Eur J Nucl Med Mol Imaging 2006;33(2):148–55.
41. Coburn NG. Lymph nodes and gastric cancer. J Surg Oncol 2009;99(4): 199–206.
42. Kim AY, Han JK, Seong CK, et al. MRI in staging advanced gastric cancer: is it useful compared with spiral CT? J Comput Assist Tomogr 2000;24(3):389–94.
43. Motohara T, Semelka RC. MRI in staging of gastric cancer. Abdom Imaging 2002;27(4):376–83.
44. Tatsumi Y, Tanigawa N, Nishimura H, et al. Preoperative diagnosis of lymph node metastases in gastric cancer by magnetic resonance imaging with ferumoxtran-10. Gastric Cancer 2006;9(2):120–8.
45. Shoda H, Kakugawa Y, Saito D, et al. Evaluation of 18F-2-deoxy-2-fluoroglucose positron emission tomography for gastric cancer screening in asymptomatic individuals undergoing endoscopy. Br J Cancer 2007;97(11): 1493–8.
46. Kwee RM, Kwee TC. Imaging in local staging of gastric cancer: a systematic review. J Clin Oncol 2007;25(15):2107–16.
47. Ganpathi IS, So JB, Ho KY. Endoscopic ultrasonography for gastric cancer: does it influence treatment? Surg Endosc 2006;20(4):559–62.
48. Jones DB. Role of endoscopic ultrasound in staging upper gastrointestinal cancers. ANZ J Surg 2007;77(3):166–72.
49. Byrne MF, Jowell PS. Gastrointestinal imaging: endoscopic ultrasound. Gastroenterology 2002;122(6):1631–48.
50. Kwee RM, Kwee TC. Imaging in assessing lymph node status in gastric cancer. Gastric Cancer 2009;12(1):6–22.

51. Coburn NG, Swallow CJ, Kiss A, et al. Significant regional variation in adequacy of lymph node assessment and survival in gastric cancer. Cancer 2006;107(9): 2143–51.
52. Schwarz RE, Smith DD. Clinical impact of lymphadenectomy extent in resectable gastric cancer of advanced stage. Ann Surg Oncol 2007;14(2):317–28.
53. Smith DD, Schwarz RR, Schwarz RE. Impact of total lymph node count on staging and survival after gastrectomy for gastric cancer: data from a large US-population database. J Clin Oncol 2005;23(28):7114–24.
54. Wagner PK, Ramaswamy A, Ruschoff J, et al. Lymph node counts in the upper abdomen: anatomical basis for lymphadenectomy in gastric cancer. Br J Surg 1991;78(7):825–7.
55. Lee SY, Hwang I, Park YS, et al. Metastatic lymph node ratio in advanced gastric carcinoma: a better prognostic factor than number of metastatic lymph nodes? Int J Oncol 2010;36(6):1461–7.
56. Sianesi M, Bezer L, Del Rio P, et al. The node ratio as prognostic factor after curative resection for gastric cancer. J Gastrointest Surg 2010;14(4):614–9.
57. Persiani R, Rausei S, Biondi A, et al. Ratio of metastatic lymph nodes: impact on staging and survival of gastric cancer. Eur J Surg Oncol 2008;34(5):519–24.
58. Japanese Gastric Cancer A. Japanese classification of gastric carcinoma - 2nd English edition. Gastric Cancer 1998;1(1):10–24.
59. Maehara Y, Hasuda S, Koga T, et al. Postoperative outcome and sites of recurrence in patients following curative resection of gastric cancer. Br J Surg 2000; 87(3):353–7.
60. Yoo CH, Noh SH, Shin DW, et al. Recurrence following curative resection for gastric carcinoma. Br J Surg 2000;87(2):236–42.
61. Ikeguchi M, Oka A, Tsujitani S, et al. Relationship between area of serosal invasion and intraperitoneal free cancer cells in patients with gastric cancer. Anticancer Res 1994;14(5B):2131–4.
62. Suzuki T, Ochiai T, Hayashi H, et al. Peritoneal lavage cytology findings as prognostic factor for gastric cancer. Semin Surg Oncol 1999;17(2):103–7.
63. Burke EC, Karpeh MS Jr, Conlon KC, et al. Peritoneal lavage cytology in gastric cancer: an independent predictor of outcome. Ann Surg Oncol 1998;5(5):411–5.
64. Hirono M, Matsuki K, Nakagami K, et al. Comparative studies on cytological and histological evaluations of disseminating peritoneal metastasis in gastric cancer. Jpn J Surg 1981;11(5):330–6.
65. Iitsuka Y, Shiota S, Matsui T, et al. Relationship between the cytologic characteristics of intraperitoneal free cancer cells and the prognosis in patients with gastric cancer. Acta Cytol 1990;34(3):437–42.
66. Fujimura T, Ohta T, Kitagawa H, et al. Trypsinogen expression and early detection for peritoneal dissemination in gastric cancer. J Surg Oncol 1998;69(2): 71–5.
67. La Torre M, Ferri M, Giovagnoli MR, et al. Peritoneal wash cytology in gastric carcinoma. Prognostic significance and therapeutic consequences. Eur J Surg Oncol 2010;36(10):982–6.
68. Makino T, Fujiwara Y, Takiguchi S, et al. The utility of pre-operative peritoneal lavage examination in serosa-invading gastric cancer patients. Surgery 2010; 148(1):96–102.
69. Bentrem D, Wilton A, Mazumdar M, et al. The value of peritoneal cytology as a preoperative predictor in patients with gastric carcinoma undergoing a curative resection. Ann Surg Oncol 2005;12(5):347–53.

70. Washington K. 7th edition of the AJCC cancer staging manual: stomach. Ann Surg Oncol 2010;17(12):3077–9.
71. Kitagawa Y, Fujii H, Mukai M, et al. The role of the sentinel lymph node in gastrointestinal cancer. Surg Clin North Am 2000;80(6):1799–809.
72. Orsenigo E, Tomajer V, Di Palo S, et al. Sentinel node mapping during laparoscopic distal gastrectomy for gastric cancer. Surg Endosc 2008;22(1):118–21.
73. Hundley JC, Shen P, Shiver SA, et al. Lymphatic mapping for gastric adenocarcinoma. Am Surg 2002;68(11):931–5.
74. Ryu KW, Lee JH, Kim HS, et al. Prediction of lymph nodes metastasis by sentinel node biopsy in gastric cancer. Eur J Surg Oncol 2003;29(10):895–9.
75. Kitagawa Y, Fujii H, Kumai K, et al. Recent advances in sentinel node navigation for gastric cancer: a paradigm shift of surgical management. J Surg Oncol 2005;90(3):147–51 [discussion: 151–2].
76. Cozzaglio L, Bottura R, Di Rocco M, et al. Sentinel lymph node biopsy in gastric cancer: possible applications and limits. Eur J Surg Oncol 2011;37(1):55–9.
77. Lee SE, Lee JH, Ryu KW, et al. Sentinel node mapping and skip metastases in patients with early gastric cancer. Ann Surg Oncol 2009;16(3):603–8.
78. Lee JH, Ryu KW, Nam BH, et al. Factors associated with detection failure and false-negative sentinel node biopsy findings in gastric cancer: results of prospective single center trials. J Surg Oncol 2009;99(3):137–42.
79. Kitagawa Y, Takeuchi H, Takagi Y, et al. Prospective multicenter trial of sentinel node mapping for gastric cancer. J Clin Oncol 2009;27:4518.
80. Rabin I, Chikman B, Lavy R, et al. The accuracy of sentinel node mapping according to T stage in patients with gastric cancer. Gastric Cancer 2010;13(1): 30–5.
81. Songun I, Bonenkamp JJ, Hermans J, et al. Prognostic value of resection-line involvement in patients undergoing curative resections for gastric cancer. Eur J Cancer 1996;32A(3):433–7.
82. Siewert JR, Bottcher K, Stein HJ, et al. Relevant prognostic factors in gastric cancer: ten-year results of the German Gastric Cancer Study. Ann Surg 1998; 228(4):449–61.
83. Sewart J, Fink U, Sendler A, et al. Gastric cancer. Curr Probl Surg 1997;34: 835–942.
84. Gouzi JL, Huguier M, Fagniez PL, et al. Total versus subtotal gastrectomy for adenocarcinoma of the gastric antrum. A French prospective controlled study. Ann Surg 1989;209(2):162–6.
85. Robertson CS, Chung SC, Woods SD, et al. A prospective randomized trial comparing R1 subtotal gastrectomy with R3 total gastrectomy for antral cancer. Ann Surg 1994;220(2):176–82.
86. Bozzetti F, Marubini E, Bonfanti G, et al. Subtotal versus total gastrectomy for gastric cancer: five-year survival rates in a multicenter randomized Italian trial. Italian Gastrointestinal Tumor Study Group. Ann Surg 1999;230(2):170–8.
87. Davies J, Johnston D, Sue-Ling H, et al. Total or subtotal gastrectomy for gastric carcinoma? A study of quality of life. World J Surg 1998;22(10):1048–55.
88. Harrison LE, Karpeh MS, Brennan MF. Proximal gastric cancers resected via a transabdominal-only approach. Results and comparisons to distal adenocarcinoma of the stomach. Ann Surg 1997;225(6):678–83 [discussion: 683–5].
89. Ohno S, Tomisaki S, Oiwa H, et al. Clinicopathologic characteristics and outcome of adenocarcinoma of the human gastric cardia in comparison with carcinoma of other regions of the stomach. J Am Coll Surg 1995;180(5):577–82.

90. Harrison LE, Karpeh MS, Brennan MF. Total gastrectomy is not necessary for proximal gastric cancer. Surgery 1998;123(2):127–30.
91. Gertler R, Rosenberg R, Feith M, et al. Pouch vs. no pouch following total gastrectomy: meta-analysis and systematic review. Am J Gastroenterol 2009; 104(11):2838–51.
92. Kurita N, Shimada M, Chikakiyo M, et al. Does Roux-en Y reconstruction with jejunal pouch after total gastrectomy prevent complications of postgastrectomy? Hepatogastroenterology 2008;55(86–87):1851–4.
93. Eypasch E, Williams JI, Wood-Dauphinee S, et al. Gastrointestinal Quality of Life Index: development, validation and application of a new instrument. Br J Surg 1995;82(2):216–22.
94. Kodama Y, Sugimachi K, Soejima K, et al. Evaluation of extensive lymph node dissection for carcinoma of the stomach. World J Surg 1981;5(2):241–8.
95. Maruyama K, Sasako M, Kinoshita T, et al. Should systematic lymph node dissection be recommended for gastric cancer? Eur J Cancer 1998;34(10):1480–9.
96. Bonenkamp JJ, Hermans J, Sasako M, et al. Extended lymph-node dissection for gastric cancer. N Engl J Med 1999;340(12):908–14.
97. Cuschieri A, Fayers P, Fielding J, et al. Postoperative morbidity and mortality after D1 and D2 resections for gastric cancer: preliminary results of the MRC randomised controlled surgical trial. The Surgical Cooperative Group. Lancet 1996;347(9007):995–9.
98. Degiuli M, Sasako M, Calgaro M, et al. Morbidity and mortality after D1 and D2 gastrectomy for cancer: interim analysis of the Italian Gastric Cancer Study Group (IGCSG) randomised surgical trial. Eur J Surg Oncol 2004;30(3):303–8.
99. Dent DM, Madden MV, Price SK. Randomized comparison of R1 and R2 gastrectomy for gastric carcinoma. Br J Surg 1988;75(2):110–2.
100. Wu CW, Hsiung CA, Lo SS, et al. Nodal dissection for patients with gastric cancer: a randomised controlled trial. Lancet Oncol 2006;7(4):309–15.
101. Wu CW, Hsiung CA, Lo SS, et al. Randomized clinical trial of morbidity after D1 and D3 surgery for gastric cancer. Br J Surg 2004;91(3):283–7.
102. de Bree E, Charalampakis V, Melissas J, et al. The extent of lymph node dissection for gastric cancer: a critical appraisal. J Surg Oncol 2010;102(6):552–62.
103. McCulloch P, Nita ME, Kazi H, et al. Extended versus limited lymph nodes dissection technique for adenocarcinoma of the stomach. Cochrane Database Syst Rev 2003;4:CD001964. PMID: 14583942; 2004;4:CD001964.
104. McCulloch P, Nita ME, Kazi H, et al. Extended versus limited lymph nodes dissection technique for adenocarcinoma of the stomach. Cochrane Database Syst Rev 2004;4:CD001964. PMID: 15495024; 2003;4:CD001964.
105. Fass J, Schumpelick V. Principles of radical surgery in gastric carcinoma. Hepatogastroenterology 1989;36(1):13–7.
106. Kwon SJ. Prognostic impact of splenectomy on gastric cancer: results of the Korean Gastric Cancer Study Group. World J Surg 1997;21(8):837–44.
107. Sugimachi K, Kodama Y, Kumashiro R, et al. Critical evaluation of prophylactic splenectomy in total gastrectomy for the stomach cancer. Gann 1980;71(5): 704–9.
108. Sakaguchi T, Sawada H, Yamada Y, et al. Indication of splenectomy for gastric carcinoma involving the proximal part of the stomach. Hepatogastroenterology 2001;48(38):603–5.
109. Bonenkamp JJ, Songun I, Hermans J, et al. Randomised comparison of morbidity after D1 and D2 dissection for gastric cancer in 996 Dutch patients. Lancet 1995;345(8952):745–8.

110. Cuschieri A, Weeden S, Fielding J, et al. Patient survival after D1 and D2 resections for gastric cancer: long-term results of the MRC randomized surgical trial. Surgical Co-operative Group. Br J Cancer 1999;79(9–10):1522–30.
111. Kasakura Y, Fujii M, Mochizuki F, et al. Is there a benefit of pancreaticosplenectomy with gastrectomy for advanced gastric cancer? Am J Surg 2000;179(3): 237–42.
112. Yu W, Choi GS, Chung HY. Randomized clinical trial of splenectomy versus splenic preservation in patients with proximal gastric cancer. Br J Surg 2006; 93(5):559–63.
113. Csendes A, Burdiles P, Rojas J, et al. A prospective randomized study comparing D2 total gastrectomy versus D2 total gastrectomy plus splenectomy in 187 patients with gastric carcinoma. Surgery 2002;131(4):401–7.
114. Kodera Y, Fujiwara M, Ohashi N, et al. Laparoscopic surgery for gastric cancer: a collective review with meta-analysis of randomized trials. J Am Coll Surg 2010; 211(5):677–86.
115. Uyama I, Sugioka A, Matsui H, et al. Laparoscopic D2 lymph node dissection for advanced gastric cancer located in the middle or lower third portion of the stomach. Gastric Cancer 2000;3(1):50–5.
116. Tanimura S, Higashino M, Fukunaga Y, et al. Laparoscopic gastrectomy for gastric cancer: experience with more than 600 cases. Surg Endosc 2008; 22(5):1161–4.
117. Kawamura H, Homma S, Yokota R, et al. Inspection of safety and accuracy of D2 lymph node dissection in laparoscopy-assisted distal gastrectomy. World J Surg 2008;32(11):2366–70.
118. Lee JH, Ryu KW, Park SR, et al. Learning curve for total gastrectomy with D2 lymph node dissection: cumulative sum analysis for qualified surgery. Ann Surg Oncol 2006;13(9):1175–81.
119. Kim HH, Hyung WJ, Cho GS, et al. Morbidity and mortality of laparoscopic gastrectomy versus open gastrectomy for gastric cancer: an interim report–a phase III multicenter, prospective, randomized Trial (KLASS Trial). Ann Surg 2010;251(3):417–20.
120. Huscher CG, Mingoli A, Sgarzini G, et al. Laparoscopic versus open subtotal gastrectomy for distal gastric cancer: five-year results of a randomized prospective trial. Ann Surg 2005;241(2):232–7.
121. Wang KK, Prasad G, Tian J. Endoscopic mucosal resection and endoscopic submucosal dissection in esophageal and gastric cancers. Curr Opin Gastroenterol 2010;26(5):453–8.
122. Eguchi T, Gotoda T, Oda I, et al. Is endoscopic one-piece mucosal resection essential for early gastric cancer? Dig Endosc 2003;15:113–6.
123. Tada M, Murakami A, Karita M, et al. Endoscopic resection of early gastric cancer. Endoscopy 1993;25(7):445–50.
124. Ida K, Nakazawa S, Yoshino J, et al. Multicentre collaborative prospective study of endoscopic treatment for early gastric cancer. Dig Endosc 2004;16:295–302.
125. Ono H, Kondo H, Gotoda T, et al. Endoscopic mucosal resection for treatment of early gastric cancer. Gut 2001;48(2):225–9.
126. Giovanni M, Berrardini D, Moutardier V, et al. Endoscopic mucosal resection (EMR): results and prognostic factors in 21 patients. Endoscopy 1999;31(9): 698–701.
127. Kojima T, Parra-Blanco A, Takahaski H, et al. Outcome of endoscopic resection for early gastric cancer: review of the Japanese literature. Gastrointest Endosc 1998;48(5):550–5.

128. Tani M, Takeshita K, Hayashi S, et al. Protection of residue or recurrence following endoscopic mucosal resection for gastric tumorous lesions. Progress of Digestive Endoscopy 1997;50:74–8.
129. Bennett C, Wang Y, Pan T. Endoscopic mucosal resection for early gastric cancer. Cochrane Database Syst Rev 2006;1:CD004276. PMID: 16437481; 2009;4:CD004276.
130. Fukase K, Kawata S. Evaluation of the efficacy of endoscopic treatment for early gastric cancer considered in terms of long-term prognosis more than 10 years - a comparison with surgical treatment. Yamagata Medical Journal 2004;22(1): 1–8.
131. Kim HS, Lee DK, Baik SK, et al. Endoscopic mucosal resection with a ligation device for early gastric cancer and precancerous lesions: comparison of its therapeutic efficacy with surgical resection. Yonsei Med J 2000;41(5):577–83.
132. Miyamoto S, Muto M, Hamamoto Y, et al. A new technique for endoscopic mucosal resection with an insulated-tip electrosurgical knife improves the completeness of resection of intramucosal gastric neoplasms. Gastrointest Endosc 2002;55(4):576–81.
133. Yamamoto H, Kawata H, Sunada K, et al. Successful en-bloc resection of large superficial tumors in the stomach and colon using sodium hyaluronate and small-caliber-tip transparent hood. Endoscopy 2003;35(8):690–4.
134. Probst A, Pommer B, Golger D, et al. Endoscopic submucosal dissection in gastric neoplasia - experience from a European center. Endoscopy 2010; 42(12):1037–44.
135. Kwee RM, Kwee TC. Predicting lymph node status in early gastric cancer. Gastric Cancer 2008;11(3):134–48.
136. Soetikno R, Kaltenbach T, Yeh R, et al. Endoscopic mucosal resection for early cancers of the upper gastrointestinal tract. J Clin Oncol 2005;23:4490–8.
137. Kaneko S, Yoshimura T. Time trend analysis of gastric cancer incidence in Japan by histological types, 1975-1989. Br J Cancer 2001;84:400–5.
138. Information Committee of the Korean Gastric Cancer Association. Nationwide gastric cancer report in Korea. J Korean Gastric Cancer Assoc 2007;7:47–54.
139. Asakuma M, Cahill RA, Lee SW, et al. NOTES: the question for minimal resection and sentinel node in early gastric cancer. World J Gastrointest Surg 2010;2(6): 203–6.
140. Cho WY, Kim YJ, Cho JY, et al. Hybrid natural orifice transluminal endoscopic surgery: endoscopic full-thickness resection of early gastric cancer and laparoscopic regional lymph node dissection - 14 human cases. Endoscopy 2011; 43(2):134–9.
141. Abe N, Takeuchi H, Yanagida O, et al. Endoscopic full-thickness resection with laparoscopic assistance as hybrid NOTES for gastric submucosal tumor. Surg Endosc 2009;23(8):1908–13.
142. Cahill RA, Asakuma M, Perretta S, et al. Gastric lymphatic mapping for sentinel node biopsy by natural orifice transluminal endoscopic surgery (NOTES). Surg Endosc 2009;23(5):1110–6.
143. Song J, Oh SJ, Kang WH, et al. Robot-assisted gastrectomy with lymph node dissection for gastric cancer: lessons learned from an initial 100 consecutive procedures. Ann Surg 2009;249(6):927–32.
144. Sano T, Sasako M, Yamamoto S, et al. Gastric cancer surgery: morbidity and mortality results from a prospective randomized controlled trial comparing D2 and extended para-aortic lymphadenectomy–Japan Clinical Oncology Group study 9501. J Clin Oncol 2004;22:2767–73.

145. Rajdev L. Treatment options for surgically resectable gastric cancer. Curr Treat Options Oncol 2010;11(1–2):14–23.
146. Lowy A, Mansfield P, Leach S, et al. Response to neoadjuvant chemotherapy best predicts survival after curative resection of gastric cancer. Ann Surg 1999;229:303–8.
147. Li W, Qin J, Sun YH, et al. Neoadjuvant chemotherapy for advanced gastric cancer: a meta-analysis. World J Gastroenterol 2010;16(44):5621–8.
148. Schuhmacher C, Schlag P, Lordick F, et al. Neoadjuvant chemotherapy versus surgery alone for locally advanced adenocarcinoma of the stomach and cardia: randomized EORTC phase III trial #40954. J Clin Oncol 2009;27(15S):4510.
149. Boige V, Pignon J, Saint-Aubert B, et al. Final results of a randomized trial comparing preoperative 5-fluorouracil (F)/cisplatin (P) to surgery alone in adenocarcinoma of stomach and lower esophagus (ASLE): FNLCC ACCORD 07-FFCD 9703 trial [abstract]. Proc Am Soc Clin Oncol 2007;25(18S):4510.
150. Cunningham D, Allum W, Stenning S, et al, MAGIC Trial Participants. Perioperative chemotherapy versus surgery alone for resectable gastroesophageal cancer. N Engl J Med 2006;355:11–20.
151. Hartgrink H, van de Velde C, Putter H, et al. Neo-adjuvant chemotherapy for operable gastric cancer: long term results of the Dutch randomised FAMTX trial. Eur J Surg Oncol 2004;30(6):643–9.
152. Nio Y, Koike M, Omori H, et al. A randomized consent design trial of neoadjuvant chemotherapy with tegafur plus uracil (UFT) for gastric cancer–a single institute study. Anticancer Res 2004;24:1879–87.
153. Zhang C, Zou S, Shi D, et al. Clinical significance of preoperative regional intra-arterial infusion chemotherapy for advanced gastric cancer. World J Gastroenterol 2004;10:3070–2.
154. Kobayashi T, Kimura T. Long-term outcome of preoperative chemotherapy with 5'-deoxy-5-fluorouridine (5'-DFUR) for gastric cancer. Gan To Kagaku Ryoho 2000;27:1521–6 [in Japanese].
155. Wang X, Wu G, Zhang M, et al. A favorable impact of preoperative FPLC chemotherapy on patients with gastric cardia cancer. Oncol Rep 2000;7:241–4.
156. Lygidakis N, Sgourakis G, Aphinives P. Upper abdominal stop-flow perfusion as a neo and adjuvant hypoxic regional chemotherapy for resectable gastric carcinoma. A prospective randomized clinical trial. Hepatogastroenterology 1999;46: 2035–8.
157. Masuyama M, Taniguchi H, Takeuchi K, et al. Recurrence and survival rate of advanced gastric cancer after preoperative EAP-II intra-arterial infusion therapy. Gan To Kagaku Ryoho 1994;21:2253–5 [in Japanese].
158. Yonemura Y, Sawa T, Kinoshita K, et al. Neoadjuvant chemotherapy for high-grade advanced gastric cancer. World J Surg 1993;17:256–61 [discussion: 261–2].
159. Nishioka B, Ouchi T, Watanabe S, et al. Follow-up study of preoperative oral administration of an antineoplastic agent as an adjuvant chemotherapy in stomach cancer. Gan To Kagaku Ryoho 1982;9:1427–32 [in Japanese].
160. Kang Y, Choi D, Im Y, et al. A phase III randomized comparison of neoadjuvant chemotherapy followed by surgery versus surgery for locally advanced stomach cancer. Abstract 503 presented at the ASCO Annual Meeting. 1996. Available at: http://www.asco.org/ASCOv2/Meetings/Abstracts?&vmview=abst_detail_view&confID=29&abstractID=10042. Accessed January 10, 2011.
161. Ng K, Meyerhardt JA, Fuchs CS. Adjuvant and neoadjuvant approaches in gastric cancer. Cancer J 2007;13(3):168–74.

162. Zhang Z, Gu X, Yin W, et al. Randomized clinical trial on the combination of preoperative irradiation and surgery in the treatment of adenocarcinoma of gastric cardia (AGC)—report on 370 patients. Int J Radiat Oncol Biol Phys 1998;42:929–34.
163. Skoropad VY, Berdov BA, Mardynski YS, et al. A prospective, randomized trial of pre-operative and intraoperative radiotherapy versus surgery alone in resectable gastric cancer. Eur J Surg Oncol 2000;26(8):773–9.
164. Sauer R, Fietkau R, Wittekind C, et al. Adjuvant vs. neoadjuvant radiochemotherapy for locally advanced rectal cancer: the German trial CAO/ARO/AIO-94. Colorectal Dis 2003;5(5):406–15.
165. Sauer R, Becker H, Hohenberger W, et al. Preoperative versus postoperative chemoradiotherapy for rectal cancer. N Engl J Med 2004;351(17):1731–40.
166. Tepper J, Krasna MJ, Niedzwiecki D, et al. Phase III trial of trimodality therapy with cisplatin, fluorouracil, radiotherapy, and surgery compared with surgery alone for esophageal cancer: CALGB 9781. J Clin Oncol 2008;26(7):1086–92.
167. Walsh TN, Grennell M, Mansoor S, et al. Neoadjuvant treatment of advanced stage esophageal adenocarcinoma increases survival. Dis Esophagus 2002; 15(2):121–4.
168. Ajani J, Mansfield P, Janjan N, et al. Multi-institutional trial of preoperative chemoradiotherapy in patients with potentially resectable gastric carcinoma. J Clin Oncol 2004;22:2774–80.
169. Ajani JA, Winter K, Okawara GS, et al. Phase II trial of preoperative chemoradiation in patients with localized gastric adenocarcinoma (RTOG 9904): quality of combined modality therapy and pathologic response. J Clin Oncol 2006; 24(24):3953–8.
170. Jansen EP, Boot H, Verheij M, et al. Optimal locoregional treatment in gastric cancer. J Clin Oncol 2005;23(20):4509–17.
171. Lim L, Michael M, Mann GB, et al. Adjuvant therapy in gastric cancer. J Clin Oncol 2005;23(25):6220–32.
172. Kattan MW, Karpeh MS, Mazumdar M, et al. Postoperative nomogram for disease-specific survival after an R0 resection for gastric carcinoma. J Clin Oncol 2003;21(19):3647–50.
173. Earle C, Maroun J. Adjuvant chemotherapy after curative resection for gastric cancer in non-Asian patients: revisiting a meta-analysis of randomized trials. Eur J Cancer 1999;35:1059–64.
174. Janunger K, Hafstrom L, Glimelius B. Chemotherapy in gastric cancer: a review and updated meta-analysis. Eur J Surg Oncol 2002;168:597–608.
175. Sakuramoto S, Sasako M, Yamaguchi T, et al. Adjuvant chemotherapy for gastric cancer with S-1, an oral fluoropyrimidine. N Engl J Med 2007;357(18):1810–20.
176. Hallissey MT, Dunn JA, Ward LC, et al. The second British Stomach Cancer Group trial of adjuvant radiotherapy or chemotherapy in resectable gastric cancer: five-year follow-up. Lancet 1994;343(8909):1309–12.
177. Macdonald JS, Smalley SR, Benedetti J, et al. Chemoradiotherapy after surgery compared with surgery alone for adenocarcinoma of the stomach or gastroesophageal junction [see comments]. N Engl J Med 2001;345(10):725–30.
178. Macdonald J, Smalley S, Benedetti J, et al. Postoperative combined radiation and chemotherapy improves disease-free survival (DFS) and overall survival (OS) in resected adenocarcinoma of the stomach and gastroesophageal junction: Update of the results of Intergroup Study INT- 0116 (SWOG 9008). Presented at the Am Soc Clin Oncol Gastrointestinal Cancers Symposium [abstract 6]. San Francisco, January 22–24, 2004.

179. Kozak KR, Moody JS. The survival impact of the intergroup 0116 trial on patients with gastric cancer. Int J Radiat Oncol Biol Phys 2008;72(2):517–21.
180. Coburn NG, Guller U, Baxter NN, et al. Adjuvant therapy for resected gastric cancer–rapid, yet incomplete adoption following results of intergroup 0116 trial. Int J Radiat Oncol Biol Phys 2008;70(4):1073–80.
181. Yonemura Y, Endou Y, Sasaki T, et al. Surgical treatment for peritoneal carcinomatosis from gastric cancer. Eur J Surg Oncol 2010;36(12):1131–8.
182. Park J, Kramer B, Steinberg S, et al. Chemosensitivity testing of human colorectal carcinoma cell lines using a tetrazolium-based colorimetric assay. Cancer Res 1987;47:5875–9.
183. Verwaal V, Bruin A, Boot H, et al. 8-Year follow-up of randomized trial: cytoreduction and hyperthermic intraperitoneal chemotherapy in patients with peritoneal carcinomatosis of colorectal cancer. Ann Surg Oncol 2008;15:2633–5.
184. Yamamura Y, Ito H, Mochizuki Y, et al. Distribution of free cancer cells in the abdominal cavity suggests limitation of bursectomy as a an essential component of radical surgery for gastric cancer. Gastric Cancer 2007;10:4–8.
185. Glehen O, Gilly F, Arvieux C, et al. Peritoneal carcinomatosis from gastric cancer: a multi-institutional study of 159 patients treated by cytoreductive surgery combined with perioperative intraperitoneal chemotherapy. Ann Surg Oncol 2010;17(9):2370–7.
186. Glehen O, Schreiber V, Cotte E, et al. Cytoreductive surgery and intraperitoneal chemohyperthermia for peritoneal carcinomatosis arising from gastric cancer. Arch Surg 2004;139:20–6.
187. Yan TD, Black D, Sugarbaker PH, et al. A systematic review and meta-analysis of the randomized controlled trials on adjuvant intraperitoneal chemotherapy for resectable gastric cancer. Ann Surg Oncol 2007;14(10):2702–13.
188. Lim S, Muhs BE, Marcus SG, et al. Results following resection for stage IV gastric cancer; are better outcomes observed in selected patient subgroups? J Surg Oncol 2007;95(2):118–22.
189. Lin SZ, Tong HF, You T, et al. Palliative gastrectomy and chemotherapy for stage IV gastric cancer. J Cancer Res Clin Oncol 2008;134(2):187–92.
190. Sougioultzis S, Syrios J, Xynos ID, et al. Palliative gastrectomy and other factors affecting overall survival in stage IV gastric adenocarcinoma patients receiving chemotherapy: a retrospective analysis. Eur J Surg Oncol 2011;37(4):312–8.
191. Takiguchi N, Oda K, Suzuki H, et al. Neoadjuvant chemotherapy with 5-fluorouracil (5-FU) or low dose *cis*-platinum (CDDP) + 5-FU in the treatment of gastric carcinoma with serosal invasion. Proc Am Soc Clin Oncol 2000;19:A1178.
192. Controlled trial of adjuvant chemotherapy following curative resection for gastric cancer. The Gastrointestinal Tumor Study Group. Cancer 1982;49(6): 1116–22.
193. Higgins GA, Amadeo JH, Smith DE, et al. Efficacy of prolonged intermittent therapy with combined 5-FU and methyl-CCNU following resection for gastric carcinoma. A Veterans Administration Surgical Oncology Group report. Cancer 1983;52(6):1105–12.
194. Engstrom PF, Lavin PT, Douglass HO Jr, et al. Postoperative adjuvant 5-fluorouracil plus methyl-CCNU therapy for gastric cancer patients. Eastern Cooperative Oncology Group study (EST 3275). Cancer 1985;55(9):1868–73.
195. Adjuvant treatments following curative resection for gastric cancer. The Italian Gastrointestinal Tumor Study Group. Br J Surg 1988;75(11):1100–4.
196. Coombes RC, Schein PS, Chilvers CE, et al. A randomized trial comparing adjuvant fluorouracil, doxorubicin, and mitomycin with no treatment in operable

gastric cancer. International Collaborative Cancer Group. J Clin Oncol 1990; 8(8):1362–9.
197. Estape J, Grau JJ, Lcobendas F, et al. Mitomycin C as an adjuvant treatment to resected gastric cancer. A 10-year follow-up. Ann Surg 1991;213(3):219–21.
198. Krook JE, O'Connell MJ, Wieand HS, et al. A prospective, randomized evaluation of intensive-course 5-fluorouracil plus doxorubicin as surgical adjuvant chemotherapy for resected gastric cancer. Cancer 1991;67(10):2454–8.
199. Kim JP, Kwon OJ, Oh ST, et al. Results of surgery on 6589 gastric cancer patients and immunochemosurgery as the best treatment of advanced gastric cancer. Ann Surg 1992;216(3):269–78.
200. Grau JJ, Estape J, Alcobendas F, et al. Positive results of adjuvant mitomycin-C in resected gastric cancer: a randomised trial on 134 patients. Eur J Cancer 1993;29A(3):340–2.
201. Lise M, Nitti D, Marchet A, et al. Final results of a phase III clinical trial of adjuvant chemotherapy with the modified fluorouracil, doxorubicin, and mitomycin regimen in resectable gastric cancer. J Clin Oncol 1995;13(11):2757–63.
202. Macdonald JS, Fleming TR, Peterson RF, et al. Adjuvant chemotherapy with 5-FU, adriamycin, and mitomycin-C (FAM) versus surgery alone for patients with locally advanced gastric adenocarcinoma: a Southwest Oncology Group study. Ann Surg Oncol 1995;2(6):488–94.
203. Neri B, Cini G, Andreoli F, et al. Randomized trial of adjuvant chemotherapy versus control after curative resection for gastric cancer: 5-year follow-up [see comments]. Br J Cancer 2001;84(7):878–80.
204. Nakajima T, Nashimoto A, Kitamura M, et al. Adjuvant mitomycin and fluorouracil followed by oral uracil plus tegafur in serosa-negative gastric cancer: a randomised trial. Gastric Cancer Surgical Study Group. Lancet 1999;354(9175): 273–7.
205. Bajetta E, Buzzoni R, Mariani L, et al. Adjuvant chemotherapy in gastric cancer: 5-year results of a randomised study by the Italian Trials in Medical Oncology (ITMO) Group. Ann Oncol 2002;13(2):299–307.
206. Nashimoto A, Nakajima T, Furukawa H, et al. Randomized trial of adjuvant chemotherapy with mitomycin, fluorouracil, and cytosine arabinoside followed by oral fluorouracil in serosa-negative gastric cancer: Japan Clinical Oncology Group 9206-1. J Clin Oncol 2003;21(12):2282–7.
207. Popiela T, Kulig J, Czupryna A, et al. Efficiency of adjuvant immunochemotherapy following curative resection in patients with locally advanced gastric cancer. Gastric Cancer 2004;7(4):240–5.
208. Bouché O, Ychou M, Burtin P, et al. Adjuvant chemotherapy with 5-fluorouracil and cisplatin compared with surgery alone for gastric cancer: 7-year results of the FFCD randomized phase III trial (8801). Ann Oncol 2005;16(9):1488–97.
209. Nitti D, Wils J, Dos Santos JG, et al. Randomized phase III trials of adjuvant FAMTX or FEMTX compared with surgery alone in resected gastric cancer. A combined analysis of the EORTC GI Group and the ICCG. Ann Oncol 2006; 17(2):262–9.
210. Nakajima T, Kinoshita T, Nashimoto A, et al. Randomized controlled trial of adjuvant uracil-tegafur versus surgery alone for serosa-negative, locally advanced gastric cancer. Br J Surg 2007;94(12):1468–76.
211. De Vita F, Giuliani F, Orditura M, et al. Adjuvant chemotherapy with epirubicin, leucovorin, 5-fluorouracil and etoposide regimen in resected gastric cancer patients: a randomized phase III trial by the Gruppo Oncologico Italia Meridionale (GOIM 9602 Study). Ann Oncol 2007;18(8):1354–8.

212. Cascinu S, Labianca R, Barone C, et al. Adjuvant treatment of high-risk, radically resected gastric cancer patients with 5-fluorouracil, leucovorin, cisplatin, and epidoxorubicin in a randomized controlled trial. J Natl Cancer Inst 2007; 99(8):601–7.
213. Di Costanzo F, Gasperoni S, Manzione L, et al. Adjuvant chemotherapy in completely resected gastric cancer: a randomized phase III trial conducted by GOIRC. J Natl Cancer Inst 2008;100(6):388–98.
214. Kulig J, Kolodziejczyk P, Sierzega M, et al. Adjuvant chemotherapy with etoposide, adriamycin and cisplatin compared with surgery alone in the treatment of gastric cancer: a phase III randomized, multicenter, clinical trial. Oncology 2010;78(1):54–61.
215. Hermans J, Bonenkamp JJ, Boon MC, et al. Adjuvant therapy after curative resection for gastric cancer: meta-analysis of randomized trials. J Clin Oncol 1993;11(8):1441–7.
216. Mari E, Floriani I, Tinazzi A, et al. Efficacy of adjuvant chemotherapy after curative resection for gastric cancer: a meta-analysis of published randomised trials. A study of the GISCAD (Gruppo Italiano per lo Studio dei Carcinomi dell'Apparato Digerente). Ann Oncol 2000;11(7):837–43.
217. Panzini I, Gianni L, Fattori PP, et al. Adjuvant chemotherapy in gastric cancer: a meta-analysis of randomized trials and a comparison with previous meta-analyses. Tumori 2002;88(1):21–7.

Gastrointestinal Stromal Tumor Surgery and Adjuvant Therapy

Valerie P. Grignol, MD[a], Paula M. Termuhlen, MD[b,*]

KEYWORDS

- GIST • Gastrointestinal stromal tumor • KIT • PDGFRA
- Imatinib mesylate

Gastrointestinal stromal tumors (GISTs) are the most common mesenchymal tumors of the gastrointestinal tract and represent 1% to 2% of all gastrointestinal malignancies. They can occur anywhere throughout the gastrointestinal tract and are seen most commonly in the stomach (60%) and small bowel (30%). They constitute 2% of gastric malignancies and 14% of tumors found in the small intestine. Overall, they are rare tumors with an annual incidence of 3000 to 5000 cases per year.[1]

The median age at presentation is 60 years with a slight male predominance. The most common symptoms at presentation are bleeding and abdominal pain. Other symptoms include dyspepsia and early satiety. GISTs are commonly found incidentally during radiologic imaging, endoscopy, and surgery.

Previously thought to be smooth muscle tumors in the class of leiomyomas and leiomyosarcomas, recent pathologic examination has noted mixed neural and myogenic features, leading them to be separately classified as GIST. They are thought to arise from the interstitial cells of Cajal, which are known as the pacemaker cells of the gut. GISTs are characterized by more than 95% being KIT (CD117)-positive. Most are composed of uniform spindle cells (70%), a small fraction are dominated by epithelioid cells, and the remaining tumors are a mix of spindle and epithelioid cells.[2]

DIAGNOSIS

GISTs are often diagnosed after resection of an undiagnosed mass and pathologic examination. In Japan, where routine screening upper gastrointestinal endoscopy is performed, many are found in early stages. The recommended evaluation for

The authors have nothing to disclose.
[a] Department of Surgery, Wright State University Boonshoft School of Medicine, Miami Valley Hospital, One Wyoming Street, WCHE 7000, Dayton, OH 45409, USA
[b] Division of Surgical Oncology, Department of Surgery, Wright State University Boonshoft School of Medicine, Miami Valley Hospital, One Wyoming Street, WCHE 7000, Dayton, OH 45409, USA
* Corresponding author.
E-mail address: Ptermuhlen9@gmail.com

Surg Clin N Am 91 (2011) 1079–1087
doi:10.1016/j.suc.2011.06.007
surgical.theclinics.com
0039-6109/11/$ – see front matter © 2011 Elsevier Inc. All rights reserved.

a gastrointestinal mass suspicious for a GIST includes CT of the chest, abdomen, and pelvis. On this imaging, the mass appears as well circumscribed and predominately extraluminal. Characteristically, GISTs have a heterogeneously enhancing soft-tissue rim surrounding a necrotic center.[3] Other examinations to consider are positron emission testing, endoscopy, and endoscopic ultrasound (EUS). EUS has been particularly useful to evaluate these subepithelial lesions and for biopsy if necessary. Percutaneous biopsy is not recommended because of the risk of rupturing the tumor and seeding the peritoneal cavity. Tissue confirmation of diagnosis is recommended only if neoadjuvant imatinib is being considered because of unresectability, or if the differential of the mass includes lymphoma.[4]

STAGING OF GIST

All GISTs are believed to have malignant potential except perhaps those smaller than 1 cm. Size and numbers of mitoses per 50 high-power fields (HPF) are the best prognostic indicators for determining the malignant potential of GISTs. Multiple staging systems for GISTs have been proposed. Besides size and mitoses, other proposed risk factors include site, evidence of tumor rupture, grade, and *KIT* mutational status.[1,5] Using EUS, the characteristics of tumor size, extraluminal border, depth, and heterogeneity have been used to predict the malignant potential of GISTs.[6] However, the criteria proposed by Miettinen and Lasota[7] at the Air Force Institute of Pathology (AFIP) may be considered the current standard for prediction. Miettinen and colleagues reviewed more than 2000 GISTs from multiple anatomic sites, with long-term follow-up, and found size, number of mitoses, and anatomic location were the most important predictors of metastatic potential. A risk stratification system was developed using their findings classifying GISTs on a spectrum from no malignant potential to high. Overall, tumors 5 cm or smaller with five or fewer mitoses per 50 HPF in the gastric location have the least malignant potential, and intestinal GISTs greater than 5 cm with more than five mitoses have the greatest malignant potential. The new Union for International Cancer Control TNM staging system closely parallels the AFIP system.[5] However, variability in reporting remains. Current studies support the need for a standardized approach to histopathologic evaluation and reporting of GIST specimens to improve risk classifications and subsequent treatment recommendations.

IMMUNOPHENOTYPING AND GENE EXPRESSION PROFILING

More than 95% of GISTs are positive for the tyrosine kinase receptor protein KIT, which is detected by the antibody CD117. Other common markers are CD34 (60%–70% of GISTs) and smooth muscle actin (SMA) (30%–40%). They are typically negative for desmin and S-100 (<5% positive).[1] In contrast, leiomyomas and leiomyosarcomas are positive for SMA and desmin, and negative for KIT and CD34, which helps distinguish GISTs from other mesenchymal tumors. However, KIT positivity may be seen in metastatic melanoma, angiosarcomas, and other tumors, although other immunotyping often can determine the true histopathology. GISTs can be KIT-negative approximately 5% of the time, making diagnosis particularly challenging.[8]

Because of the ubiquitous KIT positivity among GISTs, whether the level of expression of KIT or the presence of other proteins impacts prognosis is unknown. A retrospective study of 106 patients treated with imatinib mesylate found that expression of KIT, CD34, desmin, and S-100 had no prognostic significance in patients with GISTs.[9]

Gene expression profiling of GISTs has shown that untreated tumors have a distinct homogeneous signature that clusters separately from other sarcomas.[10,11] Signatures vary by anatomic site, with gastric GISTs having a similar signature to rectal, but small intestinal GISTs appearing much different.[11] The National Comprehensive Cancer Network (NCCN) GIST task force recently stated that gene profiling remains an investigational tool but may be useful in identifying molecular targets of tumor progression, predicting response to tyrosine kinase inhibitor therapy, and studying pathogenesis.[8]

MUTATIONS

Activating mutations of exon 11 are the most common mutations of the *KIT* receptor gene. Others include exons 9, 13, and 17.[7] Patients without *KIT* mutations often have mutations of the *PDGFR-α* receptor (PDGFRA) gene that are strongly associated with gastric GISTs and epithelioid morphology. *KIT* and *PDGFRA* mutations are mutually exclusive and found in 80% to 90% of adult GISTs. In the small cohort of patients who do not have *KIT* receptor mutations, *PDGFRA* mutations are often found. Some of the high-risk intestinal GISTs that lack either the *KIT* and *PDGFRA* mutation have been found to have a *BRAF* mutation.[12] GISTs without a mutation in either the *KIT* or *PDGFRA* genes are known as wild-type.[13] The clinical significance of the variety of mutations found in GIST has prompted much investigation.

A recent study that evaluated the prognostic significance of these mutations in 127 patients after primary resection of localized GISTs found point mutations and insertions in *KIT* exon 11 had a statistically significant favorable prognosis, whereas deletions had a worse prognosis and exon 9 mutations had a poor prognosis on univariate analysis. However, on multivariate analysis these findings were not significant.[14] Notably, exon 9 mutations are fairly specific to intestinal GISTs, which have a higher risk for progressive disease based on multiple factors.[7]

The presence and type of *KIT* mutations have been found to predict response to tyrosine kinase inhibitors in recent multiinstitutional trials. Patients with exon 11 mutations have better objective response rate (63%–83.5%) and increased progression-free survival than those with exon 9 mutations (34%–48% objective response rate) or wild-type mutations (23%–37% objective response rate).[15–17] However, for those with imatinib resistance or intolerance, GISTs with exon 9 or wild-type mutations had improved responses and progression-free survival to second-line sunitinib than those with exon 11 mutations.[15]

TREATMENT OF GIST

Management of GIST requires a multidisciplinary team, including surgeons, medical oncologists, pathologists, and radiologists. Often GISTs are identified after resection of an undiagnosed gastrointestinal mass. Thus, surgeons must be aware of the basic tenets of primary surgical treatment.

The treatment of primary, localized GISTs is surgical resection with negative margins. The morbidity is low for tumors smaller than 10 cm confined to the primary organ, and these can often be removed by a wedge or segmental resection. Lymphadenectomy is not required because these tumors rarely metastasize to the lymph nodes. The most important technical point is to avoid rupture during removal, because it increases the risk of dissemination and recurrence. GISTs are soft, friable tumors and care should be taken when handling to prevent violating the pseudocapsule. A grossly negative margin is all that is required, because microscopically positive margins have not been shown to affect survival, and management should be individualized in terms of re-resection.[18] GISTs located in the proximal stomach, especially on the greater curvature, may be amenable to wedge resection. For larger tumors, wedge resection might impact the capacitance function of the stomach and result in esophageal reflux. Surgical judgment and awareness of the gastrointestinal problems associated with extensive proximal gastrectomy are required to distinguish when wedge resection can be used as an alternative to a more formal extensive gastrectomy. After primary resection, the 5-year disease-free survival is 96% for patients with low-risk features, 54% for intermediate-risk, and 20% for high-risk.[4] The median time for recurrence is 19 to 25 months.[1]

LAPAROSCOPIC RESECTION OF GIST

Because microscopically negative margins seem to be less important in determining survival and lymph node staging is unnecessary given the rarity of lymph node metastases, the role of laparoscopy in GIST surgery has increased. Previously, only GISTs less than 2 cm in diameter were considered safe for laparoscopy. Although no large prospective trials have been performed, several case series have defined the safety and feasibility of laparoscopic resection for gastric GISTs. In two series with an average tumor size of approximately 4 cm, the 5-year disease-free survivals were 92% and 96%, respectively.[19,20] The laparoscopic approach significantly decreased length of stay and blood loss. No port site recurrences were seen. Although the patients in these studies were amenable to primary resection and overall had a low malignant potential, survival was determined by the same factors (size, mitoses) as open. Therefore, the goals of surgery for laparoscopy remain the same as those for open technique: grossly negative margins, removal of the tumor without rupture, avoidance of tumor manipulation, and following the principles of oncology. Use of a hand port is recommended as needed for larger tumors to allow for safe and intact removal, and an experienced endoscopist should be present for localization of intragastric lesions.[19] Laparoscopic resection of GIST is technically feasible and can be safely performed.

METASTATIC GIST

In 20% to 30% of patients, GISTs have already developed metastases to the viscera or the peritoneum at presentation. The most common sites of synchronous metastases or subsequent recurrence are liver, peritoneum, or both. Metastases to the lung and bone occur late. Because of the multifocality and diffuse nature of recurrence, this stage of disease is not usually amenable to surgical resection. Historically, treatment with surgery alone for metastatic GIST was associated with poor survival. However, the treatment of metastatic GIST helped to develop the concept of targeted therapy.

TYROSINE KINASE INHIBITOR THERAPY

Imatinib Mesylate

In a disease that recurs in approximately 50% of patients within 5 years and chemotherapy is ineffective, the discovery of the mutation of the *KIT* gene in 1998 and the subsequent development of imatinib mesylate, a receptor tyrosine kinase inhibitor, revolutionized the treatment of recurrent and metastatic GIST.[21–23] Imatinib is a potent selective small molecular inhibitor of a family of structurally related tyrosine kinase signaling enzymes, including KIT, the leukemia-specific BCR-ABL chimera, and PDGFRA.[8] Imatinib has shown an 80% clinical benefit in phase II trials of patients with advanced or recurrent GIST. Progression-free survival of up to 20 to 24 months has been noted with doses of 400 mg/d.[2,4] Phase III escalation trials of 800 mg/d did not show a benefit with higher doses of imatinib, except in patients with exon 9 *KIT* mutations. Therefore, a standard dose of 400 mg/d of imatinib in recommended unless the exon 9 mutation exists, and then 800 mg/d is recommended.[24] Primary resistance to imatinib can occur (ie, disease progression within 6 months of treatment). However, secondary resistance (progression after 6 months after evidence of initial effectiveness) occurs more frequently, with an average time to progression of 20 months. It is believed to occur through development of a secondary acquired *KIT* mutation.[8] Therefore, the development of other agents has been necessary.

Sunitinib Malate

The U.S. Food and Drug Administration approved sunitinib malate in 2006, another small molecule inhibitor of receptor tyrosine kinases that has been shown to be an effective second-line therapy for patients with GISTs.[2,25,26] Sunitinib is believed to bind to different kinases thought to cause aberrant behavior of GIST, and has particular effectiveness in patients who have GISTs with the exon 9 mutation.[15] In a randomized, placebo-controlled, double-blind study of patients with unresectable imatinib-resistant GIST, time to tumor progression improved from 6.4 weeks in the placebo arm to 27.3 weeks in the sunitinib group.[27] Some findings also suggest that imatinib-resistant recurrent disease may respond better to sunitinib after cytoreductive surgery.[28] As more is understood about the molecular biology of GISTs, new targeted therapies are being developed.

ADJUVANT TREATMENT OF RESECTED GIST

The benefit of imatinib mesylate in the adjuvant setting has been shown in phase III randomized controlled trials. The recently completed Z9000 and Z9001 trials conducted by the American College of Surgeons Oncology Group (ACOSOG) showed that imatinib provides benefit in patients with intermediate to high risk (nongastric and/or large tumors) that have KIT-positive GIST. A dose of 400 mg/d of imatinib for a year is the recommended treatment.[29] However, controversy over the duration of therapy remains, with future trials being designed to answer this question.[8,30]

NEOADJUVANT TREATMENT OF GIST

Several clinical trials have recently been completed evaluating the efficacy of imatinib in unresectable or marginally resectable disease. Although these studies involved small numbers of patients, tumor size reduction and improved respectability were observed.[31] Despite the limited data, imatinib is the preferred initial treatment for patients with locally advanced unresectable disease. However, until more confirmatory work is performed, the use of imatinib in the neoadjuvant setting for radiographically resectable disease remains investigational and is not currently recommended.

SURGICAL TREATMENT OF METASTATIC GIST

Imatinib is the standard for treating recurrent or metastatic GIST. However, because it is associated with a median time to recurrence of less than 2 years, surgical resection in patients with residual disease has been considered. Some patients may benefit from surgical resection of remaining gross disease to improve progression-free survival and prevent secondary resistance, because remaining tumor harbor cells are capable of undergoing mutation and are the clones presumed resistant to therapy.[32] Resection should include removal of all gross disease and may require multivisceral resection, omentectomy, and peritoneal stripping. Because liver metastases are often multicentric and not amenable to traditional segmental or lobar hepatectomy, radiofrequency ablation or hepatic embolization can be performed. Surgical therapy may be especially appropriate for patients who do not have access to clinical trials to receive further medical therapy.[8]

PEDIATRIC GIST

Although rare in children, 1% to 2% of GISTs do occur in the pediatric population and are thought to be fundamentally different entities from adult GISTs. These GISTs typically lack *KIT* and *PDGFRA* mutations (wild-type GIST) and strongly express CD117. Pediatric wild-type GISTs have different characteristics from adult wild-type GISTs. A recent study suggested that defects in succinate dehydrogenase may be the impetus for oncogenesis in patients affected by pediatric GIST. Testing for germline mutations in succinate dehydrogenase has been recommended in this population.[33] Pediatric GISTs, unlike adult sporadic GISTs, metastasize to the lymph nodes and are more commonly epithelioid. They are almost exclusively gastric in origin and, unlike adult GISTs, are more common in girls. Surgery with repeat resections for recurrence is the mainstay of therapy because response to tyrosine kinase inhibitor therapy may be limited. The NCCN GIST task force recommended that pediatric patients with GIST be referred to specialty centers or treated in the context of clinical trials, because of the unique nature of the tumors.[8] The National Institutes of Health organized a consortium for pediatric GIST research (http://www.pediatricgist.cancer.gov/CPGR).

GIST ASSOCIATED WITH OTHER TUMORS AND SYNDROMES

A rare entity that resembles pediatric GIST but is more commonly found in women is known as Carney triad. Patients have multifocal gastric GISTs, paragangliomas, and pulmonary chondromas.[34] The clinical course can be prolonged even in the face of lymph node or visceral metastases. Carney-Stratakis syndrome is characterized by the presence of a GIST and paragangliomas.

Inherited germline mutations in either *KIT* or *PDGFRA* produce familial GISTs. Associated clinical findings of hyperpigmentation and gastrointestinal dysfunction, such as dysphagia or irritable bowel syndrome, are commonly present. Age of onset is typically in the fifth decade and 90% of patients develop a GIST by 70 years of age. Most familial GISTs have favorable histologic features, and patients do not have a shortened survival if affected.[35–37]

GISTs are one of the malignancies seen in association with neurofibromatosis-1. Age at presentation is similar to that for adult sporadic GIST, but tumors are more commonly found in the small intestine. Imatinib seems to have limited effect in these patients, and many experience progression, with a median survival of 21 months.[38]

SUMMARY

GISTs are a unique class of mesenchymal tumors specifically identified within the past decade. Intense molecular and genetic study has been used to characterize these tumors and develop treatment strategies. Although the mainstay of treatment remains surgical resection, therapy targeted at the inhibition of tyrosine kinases has had dramatic results. Because of the rapid accumulation of information about the diagnosis and treatment of these tumors, the NCCN convened a GIST task force to provide updated recommendations in 2010. As understanding of these tumors advances, rapid changes in treatment recommendations will continue and should warrant regular updates in tumor management.

REFERENCES

1. Gold JS, DeMatteo RP. Combined surgical and molecular therapy: the gastrointestinal stromal model. Ann Surg 2006;244:176–84.

2. Coffey RJ, Washington MK, Corless CL, et al. Ménétrier disease and gastrointestinal stromal tumors: hyperproliferative disorders of the stomach. J Clin Invest 2007;117:70–80.
3. Burkhill GJ, Badran M, Al-Muderis O, et al. Malignant gastrointestinal stromal tumor: distribution, imaging features, and pattern of metastatic spread. Radiology 2003;226:527–32.
4. Deshaies I, Cherenfant J, Gusani NJ, et al. Gastrointestinal stromal tumor (GIST) recurrence following surgery: review of the clinical utility of imatinib treatment. Ther Clin Risk Manag 2010;6:453–8.
5. Agaimy A. Gastrointestinal stromal tumors (GIST) from risk stratification systems to the new TNM proposal: more questions than answers? A review emphasizing the need for a standardized GIST reporting. Int J Clin Exp Pathol 2010;3:461–71.
6. Shah P, Gao F, Edmundowicz SA, et al. Predicting malignant potential of gastrointestinal stromal tumors using endoscopic ultrasound. Dig Dis Sci 2009;54:1265–9.
7. Miettinen M, Lasota J. Gastrointestinal stromal tumors. Arch Pathol Lab Med 2006;130:1466–78.
8. Demetri GD, von Mehren M, Antonescu CR, et al. NCCN task force report: update on the management of patients with gastrointestinal stromal tumors. J Natl Compr Canc Netw 2010;8(Suppl 2):S1–41.
9. Chirieac LR, Trent JC, Steinert DM, et al. Correlation of immunophenotype with progression-free survival in patients with gastrointestinal stromal tumors treated with imatinib mesylate. Cancer 2006;107:2237–44.
10. Nielsen TO, West RB, Linn SC, et al. Molecular characterisation of soft tissue tumours: a gene expression study. Lancet 2002;359:1301–7.
11. Antonescu CR, Viale A, Sarran L, et al. Gene expression in gastrointestinal stromal is distinguished by KIT genotype and anatomic site. Clin Cancer Res 2004;10:3282–90.
12. Agaram NP, Wong GC, Guo T, et al. Novel V600E BRAF mutations in imatinib-naïve and imatinib-resistant gastrointestinal stromal tumors. Genes Chromosomes Cancer 2008;47:853–9.
13. Lasota J, Miettinen M. Clinical significance of oncogenic KIT and PDGFRA mutations in gastrointestinal stromal tumours. Histopathology 2008;53:245–66.
14. DeMatteo RP, Gold JS, Saran L, et al. Tumor mitotic rate, size, and location independently predict recurrence after resection of primary gastrointestinal stromal tumor (GIST). Cancer 2008;112:608–15.
15. Heinrich MC, Maki RG, Corless CL, et al. Primary and secondary kinase genotypes correlate with the biological and clinical activity of sunitinib in imatinib-resistant gastrointestinal stromal tumor. J Clin Oncol 2008;26:5352–9.
16. Heinrich MC, Owzar K, Corless CL, et al. Correlation of kinas genotype and clinical outcome in the North American Intergroup phase III trial of imatinib mesylate for treatment of advanced gastrointestinal stromal tumor: CALGB 150105 Study by Cancer and Leukemia Group B and Southwest Oncology Group. J Clin Oncol 2008;26:5360–7.
17. Debiec-Rychter M, Sciot R, Le Cesne A, et al. KIT mutations and dose selection for imatinib in patients with advanced gastrointestinal stromal tumours. Eur J Cancer 2006;42:1093–103.
18. DeMatteo RP, Lewis JJ, Leung D, et al. Two hundred gastrointestinal stromal tumors: recurrence patterns and prognostic factors for survival. Ann Surg 2000;231:51–8.

19. Novitsky YW, Kercher KW, Sing RF, et al. Long-term outcomes of laparoscopic resection of gastrointestinal stromal tumors. Ann Surg 2006;243:738–45.
20. Otani Y, Furukawa T, Yoshida M, et al. Operative indications for relatively small (2–5cm) gastrointestinal stromal tumor of the stomach based on analysis of 60 operated cases. Surgery 2006;139:484–92.
21. Hirota S, Isozaki K, Moriyama Y, et al. Gain-of-function mutations of c-kit in human gastrointestinal stromal tumors. Science 1998;279:577–80.
22. Joensuu H, Roberts PJ, Sarlomo-Rikala M, et al. Effect of the tyrosine kinase inhibitor STI571 in a patient with a metastatic gastrointestinal stromal tumor. N Engl J Med 2001;344:1052–6.
23. DeMatteo RP, Heinrich MC, ElRifai WM, et al. Clinical management of gastrointestinal stromal tumors: before and after STI-571. Hum Pathol 2002;33:466–77.
24. Gastrointestinal Stromal Tumor Meta-Analysis Group. Comparison of two doses of imatinib for the treatment of unresectable or metastatic gastrointestinal stromal tumors: a meta-analysis of 1640 patients. J Clin Oncol 2010;28:1247–53.
25. Younus J, Verma S, Franek J, et al. Sunitinib malate for gastrointestinal stromal tumour in imatinib mesylate-resistant patients: recommendations and evidence. Curr Oncol 2010;17:4–10.
26. Blay JY, von Mehren M, Blackstein ME. Perspective on updated treatment guidelines for patients with gastrointestinal stromal tumors. Cancer 2010;116:5126–37.
27. Demetri GD, van Oosterom AT, Garrett CR, et al. Efficacy and safety of sunitinib in patients with advanced gastrointestinal stromal tumour after failure of imatinib: a randomized controlled trial. Lancet 2006;368:1329–38.
28. Raut CP, Wang Q, Manola J, et al. Cytoreductive surgery in patients with metastatic gastrointestinal stromal tumor treated with sunitinib malate. Ann Surg Oncol 2010;17:407–15.
29. DeMatteo RP, Ballman KV, Antonescu CR, et al. Adjuvant imatinib mesylate after resection of localised, primary gastrointestinal stromal tumour: a randomised, double-blind, placebo-controlled trial. Lancet 2009;373:1097–104.
30. Blay JY. A decade of tyrosine kinase inhibitor therapy: historical and current perspectives on targeted therapy for GIST. Cancer Treat Rev 2011;37(5):373–84.
31. Sjolund K, Andersson A, Nilsson E, et al. Downsizing treatment with tyrosine kinase inhibitors in patients with advanced gastrointestinal stromal tumors improved resectability. World J Surg 2010;34:2090–7.
32. Yeh CN, Chen TW, Tseng JH, et al. Surgical management in metastatic gastrointestinal stromal tumor (GIST) patients after imatinib mesylate treatment. J Surg Oncol 2010;102:599–603.
33. Janeway KA, Kim SY, Lodish M, et al. Defects in succinate dehydrogenase in gastrointestinal stromal tumors lacking KT and PDGFRA mutations. Proc Natl Acad Sci U S A 2011;108:314–8.
34. Stratakis CA, Carney JA. The triad of paragangliomas, gastric stromal tumours and pulmonary chondromas (Carney triad), and the dyad of paragangliomas and gastric stromal sarcomas (Carney-Stratakis syndrome): molecular genetics and clinical implications. J Intern Med 2009;266:43–52.
35. Kleinbaum EP, Lazar AJ, Tamborini E, et al. Clinical, histopathologic, molecular and therapeutic findings in a large kindred with gastrointestinal stromal tumor. Int J Cancer 2008;122:711–8.
36. Agarwal R, Robson M. Inherited predisposition to gastrointestinal stromal tumor. Hematol Oncol Clin North Am 2009;23:1–13.

37. Antonescu CR. Gastrointestinal stromal tumor (GIST) pathogenesis, familial GIST, and animal models. Semin Diagn Pathol 2006;23:63–9.
38. Mussi C, Schildhaus HU, Gronchi A, et al. Therapeutic consequences from molecular biology for gastrointestinal stromal tumor patients affected by neurofibromatosis type I. Clin Cancer Res 2008;14:4550–5.

Minimally Invasive Gastric Surgery

Alfredo M. Carbonell II, DO

KEYWORDS

• Gastric • Stomach • GIST • Stromal • Submucosal tumor
• Cancer • Ulcer • Laparoscopy

The most common indications for gastric resection remain benign ulcer disease and neoplasm. Surgery for these diseases can be performed safely with laparoscopy. As surgeons adhere to the original tenets of open gastric resections while performing laparoscopic resections, disease outcomes will remain the same with the improved surgical outcomes of less pain, shorter hospital stay, and a lower incidence of wound complications.

Laparoscopic gastric resections can be divided into the more straightforward wedge/tumor resections performed for submucosal tumors or the more formal anatomic gastric resections, such as those required for refractory ulcer disease or malignancy. This article reviews the tools and techniques for laparoscopic gastric resection.

PATIENT POSITIONING AND EQUIPMENT

Positioning

For ergonomic reasons, we perform gastric surgery standing between patients' legs. This positioning is accomplished by placing patients on a split-leg table or positioning them in the low lithotomy position in stirrups (**Fig. 1**). The patients' arms are extended, and 2 monitors are placed at the head of the table, providing excellent visualization for all members of the operating team.

Port placement varies depending on the planned anatomic resection or tumor location within the stomach. With little exception, the standard 5-port technique used for laparoscopic antireflux surgery is often sufficient (**Fig. 2**). A 5- or 10-mm port is placed at or just above the umbilicus for a 30° angled laparoscope. The surgeon uses right and left epigastric ports for the dissection and resection. These ports are 5 mm to 12 mm in size. The 12-mm port can be used for the insertion of an endoscopic stapler and the introduction of a laparoscopic ultrasound probe, if necessary. A 5-mm port is placed in the right subcostal location at the midclavicular line. A liver retractor is

The author has nothing to disclose.
Division of Minimal Access and Bariatric Surgery, Greenville Hospital System University Medical Center, University of South Carolina School of Medicine, 890 West Faris Road, Suite 310, Greenville, SC 29605, USA
E-mail address: acarbonell@ghs.org

Surg Clin N Am 91 (2011) 1089–1103
doi:10.1016/j.suc.2011.06.006 surgical.theclinics.com
0039-6109/11/$ – see front matter © 2011 Elsevier Inc. All rights reserved.

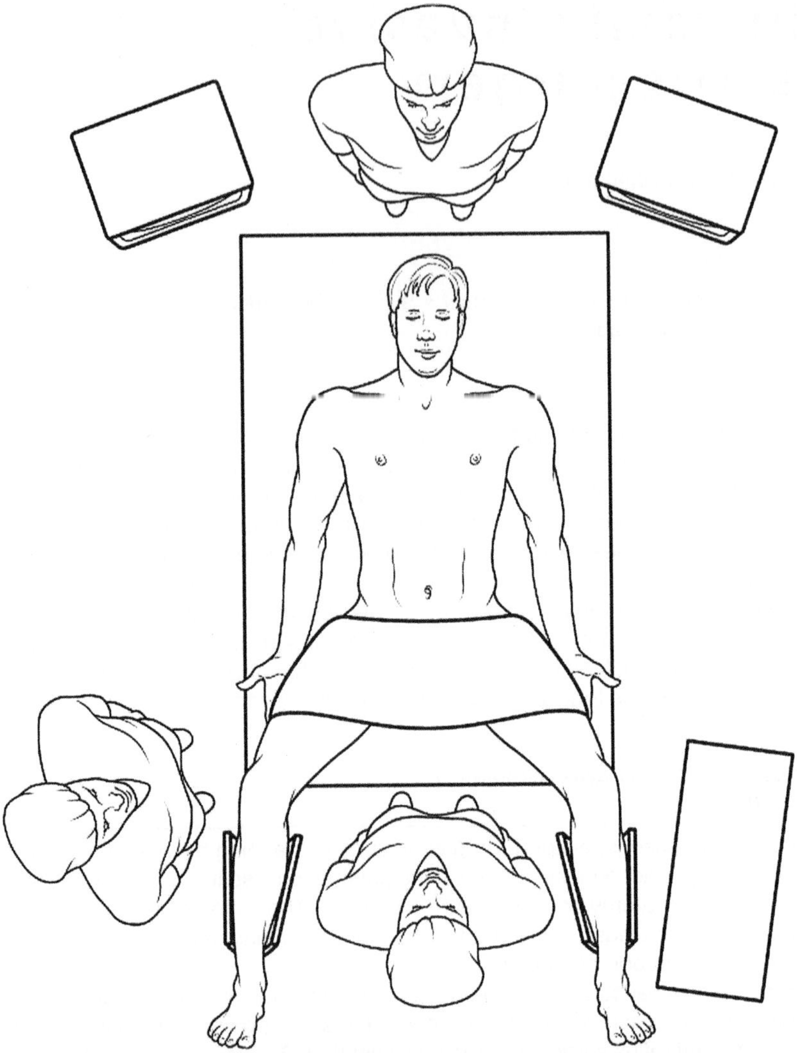

Fig. 1. Patient positioning on a split-leg table for laparoscopic gastric resection. The surgeon stands between the patient's legs and the assistants stand to each side. (*Courtesy of* B. Todd Heniford, MD, Carolinas Medical Center, Charlotte, NC.)

placed through this port to retract the left lateral hepatic segments and held in position with a laparoscopic holding device clamped to the side of the bed. An assistant's port (5 mm) is placed in the left lateral abdomen parallel to the camera port to aid in retraction and manipulation of the stomach. In the event that a formal gastric resection is required or for tumors in the lower gastric body, the aforementioned trocar setup is simply readjusted 5 cm caudal. Patients are placed in the reverse Trendelenburg position to enhance exposure of the stomach. It is recommended that some mark be made at the level of the patients' head or ear on the table to alert the anesthesiologist if patients have slid inferiorly and to allow for the correction of positioning.

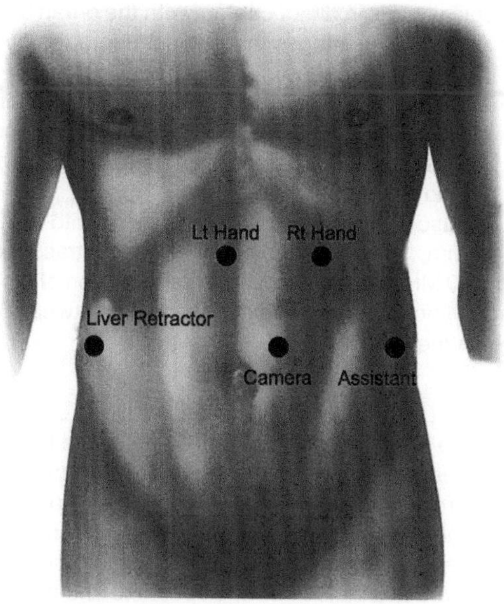

Fig. 2. The trocar configuration for laparoscopic gastric resections is similar to that of standard laparoscopic antireflux surgery.

Flexible Endoscopy

Intraoperative flexible endoscopy is a critical part of any laparoscopic gastric resection. It complements the outside laparoscopic view with an inside view of the stomach. Although computed tomography may help with tumor localization, there is no substitute for precise intraoperative endoscopic tumor localization. Preoperative endoscopy, particularly when performed by anyone other than the operating surgeon, is often misleading and may not precisely identify the tumor as being located along the anterior or posterior gastric wall. Some gastric lesions, particularly gastrointestinal stromal tumors (GIST), may have more of an intraluminal versus extraluminal component or vice versa, consequently, the operative approach may need to be adjusted. With an endoscope inside the stomach, the surgeon can palpate the edges of the lesion with instruments and obtain visual confirmation of its exact location. This maneuver is indispensable when performing gastric wedge resections because it allows for precise endoscopic stapler placement. Additionally, intraoperative endoscopy aids in the detection of anastomotic or staple line problems because the surgeon can test for air leaks at the conclusion of the procedure. In some hybrid approaches to gastric resection, tumors may even be captured in a specimen retrieval bag and removed endoscopically.

Intraoperative Laparoscopic Ultrasound

Intraoperative laparoscopic ultrasound is a dynamic imaging modality that provides interactive and timely information during surgical procedures. When used during the laparoscopic resection of submucosal tumors, it enhances tumor identification within the stomach, allows for a detailed evaluation of the liver for the possibility of metastatic disease, and guides intraoperative biopsy if necessary.[1] Because the transducer is introduced laparoscopically, it is in direct contact with the organ being examined. This position results in high-resolution images that are not degraded by air, bone, or overlying soft tissue.

Laparoscopic ultrasound can detect intrahepatic lesions or multilobar disease not visualized during routine preoperative imaging. Periportal, peripancreatic, and celiac adenopathy can be detected by laparoscopic ultrasound, although the risk of lymphatic spread is rare in GIST of the stomach.[2]

The laparoscopic ultrasound probe can be introduced into the abdomen through a 12-mm port. A 10-mm, multifrequency, articulating ultrasound probe is set at a frequency of 7.5 to 10.0 MHz to achieve optimal visualization of the superficial hepatic parenchyma. The probe should be set at low frequencies, between 5 to 7 MHz, to attain deep penetration within the liver.[3]

Instruments

Retraction of the left lobe of the liver is typically required with formal gastric resection and wedge gastrectomies of the lesser curve and anterior body. Numerous 5-mm and 10-mm liver retractors are available. The author's preferred model is the Diamond Flex retractor (Genzyme, Tucker, Georgia), and others like it, which can pass through a 5-mm cannula and form a large triangle when configured in the abdomen. Other fan-type, 10-mm retractors are available in both disposable and nondisposable forms.

Graspers are manufactured by numerous companies and are typically selected by personal preference. The author finds the use of the Dorsey bowel graspers (Karl Storz, Tuttlingen, Germany) or other such atraumatic graspers useful for intestinal manipulation because they have a large surface area with which to handle the bowel. This increased surface area allows for even distribution of shear force on the bowel wall and may help to prevent unrecognized serosal tears or enterotomies. Additional standard instruments are required, including Maryland-type dissectors, 5-mm and 10-mm laparoscopes, clip appliers, and needle drivers.

Electrosurgical Energy Sources

Should the laparoscopic gastric resection require division of the short gastric or gastroepiploic vessels, a more robust energy source capable of controlling these larger pedicles may be required. Ultrasonic coagulating shears and bipolar vessel-sealing devices available from multiple manufacturers allow for division of vessels upwards of 7 mm in diameter. The author prefers the use of ultrasonic shears because they can also be used to incise the gastric wall and resect the tumor along with some surrounding normal gastric tissue.

Staplers

The endoscopic gastrointestinal anastomosis (GIA) stapling device is perhaps the single most important piece of equipment for laparoscopic gastric resection. The endoscopic GIA staplers come with linear staple cartridge lengths of 30, 45, and 60 mm with or without articulating ends. Additionally, the staple height is important because the thickness of the stomach varies at different areas (thinner at the fundus and thicker at the body). This factor becomes important because staple height choice can play a role in staple-line bleeding and leaks. Previous investigators found a decreased staple-line bleed rate in gastric bypass when they downsized their gastric staples from 4.8 to 3.5 mm and their small bowel staples to 2.5 mm.[4] The author uses the 45 mm length, 3.5-mm staple height cartridges for transection of the gastric fundus and the small bowel and the creation of the jejunojejunostomy.

Absorbable staple-line reinforcement or buttressing has been shown by several investigators to reduce the incidence of staple-line bleeding, expedite gastric resection, and reduce circular stapled anastomotic stricture.[5,6] For these same reasons, the author prefers to use staple-line reinforcement for formal gastric resections and circular stapled anastomoses. Additionally, the remaining staple-line buttress can serve as a handle with which to manipulate the gastric pouch as needed.

WEDGE/TUMOR RESECTION TECHNIQUES

Tumors of the Anterior Wall

Submucosal tumors within the anterior wall of the stomach are amenable to wedge resection with a linear endoscopic GIA stapler. Once the tumor is identified, it can be balloted between 2 laparoscopic instruments. Wedge resection can be performed in 2 ways. First, the gastric wall near the tumor can be elevated with a bowel grasper or with traction sutures placed into normal gastric tissue above and below the lesion. This method works best for small intraluminal or mostly extraluminal tumors. The gastric wedge, which includes the tumor, is placed between the jaws of the endoscopic GIA stapler and the stapler is fired (**Fig. 3**). Typically, multiple staple firings are required to complete the wedge resection. The direction of the resection staple line is not as important on the anterior gastric wall. However, a wedge resection staple line may cause deformity of the gastric outlet when the tumor arises closer to the pylorus.

A second technique that works well for large extraluminal or large intraluminal tumors is where ultrasonic shears are used to excise the tumor along with a small surrounding rim of normal gastric tissue (**Fig. 4**). Compared with a stapled wedge resection, this technique allows for a more precise excision of normal tissue margins; however, it requires the closure of a large gastrotomy, which is a more complex task. The gastrotomy can be sutured closed intracorporeally or closed with an endoscopic GIA stapler. When using the stapler for closure the author places 2 to 4 full-thickness traction sutures along the cut edge of the gastric wall to line up the opposing sides of the gastrotomy (**Fig. 5**). This procedure aids in simplifying and ensuring a full-thickness closure. All staple and suture lines are tested by placing patients in the Trendelenburg position, submerging the stomach under saline, and insufflating air via an upper endoscope to identify any leak from the staple line.

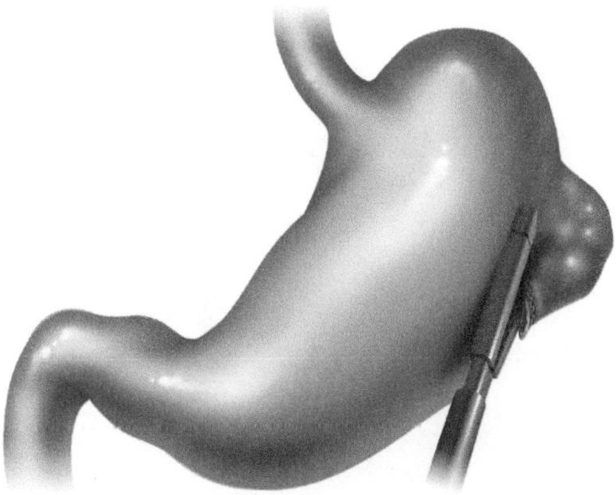

Fig. 3. Stapled wedge gastrectomy to include the submucosal tumor. (*Courtesy of* B. Todd Heniford, MD, Carolinas Medical Center, Charlotte, NC.)

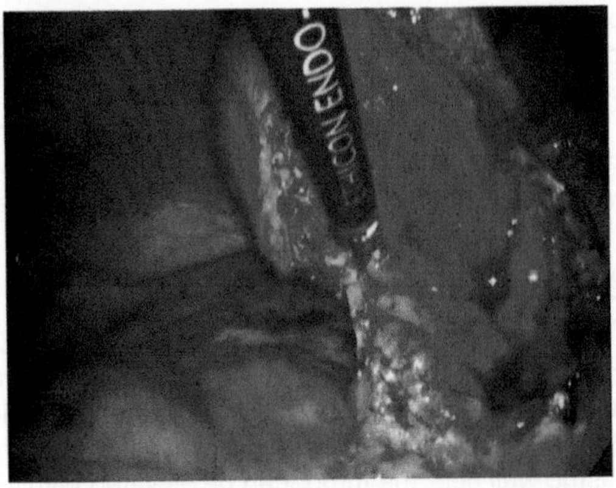

Fig. 4. Large submucosal tumor undergoing resection along with a rim of normal surrounding gastric tissue using ultrasonic shears.

Tumors of the Posterior Wall

Posterior wall tumors can be approached in several ways. If the tumor is small and intraluminal or larger but extraluminal, a stapled wedge resection as previously described can be performed. Because the tumor is located along the posterior wall, division of the short gastric vessels is required and the stomach is spiraled counter-clockwise to visualize the posterior wall.

For larger tumors that are mostly intraluminal, a second method involves creating an anterior gastrotomy over the lesion after it has been endoscopically localized within the stomach along the posterior wall. Working inside the stomach, the normal mucosal tissue adjacent to the lesion is held with traction sutures. The tumor and surrounding normal stomach is then elevated through the gastrotomy. The tumor is excised along with a margin of normal tissue using an endoscopic GIA stapler (**Fig. 6**). The staple line is observed for bleeding, and any bleeding points are oversewn. The gastrotomy is either sutured or stapled closed as previously described.

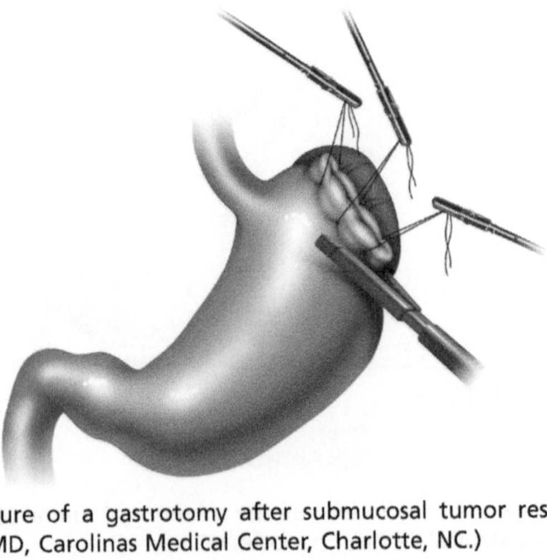

Fig. 5. Stapled closure of a gastrotomy after submucosal tumor resection. (*Courtesy of* B. Todd Heniford, MD, Carolinas Medical Center, Charlotte, NC.)

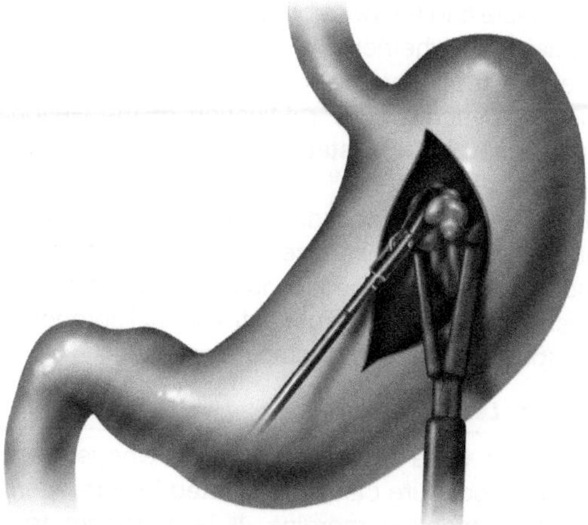

Fig. 6. Resection of posterior wall submucosal tumor through an anterior gastrotomy. (*Courtesy of* B. Todd Heniford, MD, Carolinas Medical Center, Charlotte, NC.)

A third method for smaller intraluminal tumors closer to the lesser curvature or where a stapled wedge resection may be unfeasible is the percutaneous intragastric technique (**Fig. 7**) first popularized by Ohashi[7] for early gastric cancers. This technique involves the placement of 3 dilating-type or balloon-tipped laparoscopic trocars (5–10 mm) transabdominally directly into the lumen of the insufflated stomach.[8] The lesion is identified, and a dilute epinephrine solution (1:100,000) is injected circumferentially as a tumescent to aid in the dissection of the submucosal plane and to limit bleeding. The lesion is carefully enucleated from the submucosal-muscular junction using hook cautery. The mucosal defect is left open to heal or can be closed with intragastric suturing. The tumor can be placed in a retrieval bag that is grasped endoscopically and removed transorally. The one potential pitfall of enucleation is inadvertent violation

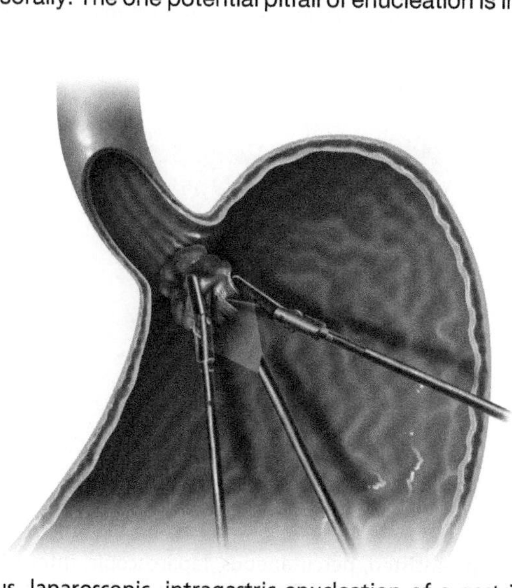

Fig. 7. Percutaneous, laparoscopic, intragastric enucleation of a gastric submucosal mass. (*Courtesy of* B. Todd Heniford, MD, Carolinas Medical Center, Charlotte, NC.)

of the tumor pseudocapsule and the possibility of leaving behind microscopic disease. With GIST, the arguments of whether it is acceptable to have microscopic positive margins versus not and resection versus enucleation for tumors in difficult locations is still debated. The most recent 2007 ratification of the National Comprehensive Cancer Network guidelines on GIST states that negative microscopic margins are the key objective of surgical treatment.[9]

Because safe resection of submucosal tumors requires that the entire lesion be resected intact, caution should be exercised when using the intragastric technique. Complete gastric mobilization is required to visualize the exterior aspect of the posterior gastric wall to ensure there is not a larger extraluminal component to the tumor that could be left behind upon enucleation or stapled resection.

Tumors of the Greater or Lesser Curvature

Tumors of the curvatures may be amenable to simple wedge resection with an endoscopic GIA stapler. This procedure can be facilitated by intraoperative endoscopy to confirm adequate gross resection margins. It is important to divide the greater omentum for greater curvature tumors and the gastrohepatic ligament for those tumors located on the lesser curve. Rolling the stomach so that the lesion faces anteriorly facilitates the resection.

Tumors of the Gastroesophageal Junction

Historically, tumors located at this extreme of the stomach required extensive gastroesophageal resection and a combined thoracoabdominal incision. Changes in gastric and esophageal function or gastric emptying after resection can be underestimated, resulting in significant disability. Heniford and colleagues[8] reported a novel approach to the gastroesophageal junction tumor using a minilaparoscopic intragastric technique (**Fig. 8**). A gastroscope serves as the camera and insufflator, and two 2-mm mushroom-tipped ports are placed transabdominally through the gastric wall to perform the resection. Hook cautery is used to enucleate the tumors adjacent to the gastroesophageal junction following a submucosal 1:100,000 epinephrine injection. The mass is then removed transorally in a specimen retrieval bag via the endoscope.

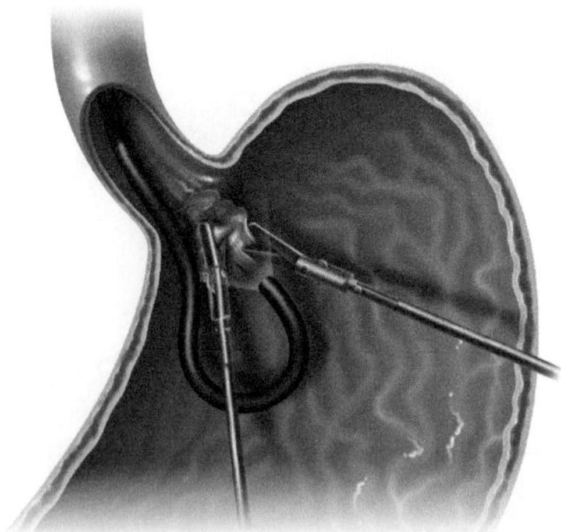

Fig. 8. Flexible endoscopic-assisted, percutaneous, laparoscopic, intragastric enucleation of a gastric submucosal mass. (*Courtesy of* B. Todd Heniford, MD, Carolinas Medical Center, Charlotte, NC.)

Alternatively, the lesion can be completely staple wedge resected intraluminally. This technique requires at least one 12-mm intraluminal trocar for introduction of the endoscopic GIA stapler. A flexible gastroscope placed slightly intragastric helps to identify and protect the gastroesophageal junction (**Fig. 9**). When using any of the intragastric resection techniques, it is important to triangulate the trocars within the stomach because the working space is extremely limited. Once the resection is complete, the small gastrotomies are simply sutured closed.

If the tumor is of significant size or has a large extraluminal component, then partial esophagogastrectomy may be required. This procedure can be performed laparoscopically; however, conversion to an open transabdominal or thoracoabdominal approach may be necessary. After division of the short gastric vessels and the lesser curve attachments, the proximal esophagus is mobilized well into the mediastinum. When an adequate length of esophagus and stomach has been dissected free, the distal esophagus, proximal to the submucosal tumor, is transected at 90° with an angled articulating 45-mm endoscopic linear stapler through a 12-mm port placed in the left upper quadrant. A second transection below the tumor, onto the stomach, is then performed. If the left gastric artery is sacrificed in this approach, it is important to transect the stomach distal to the tumor along a line from the incisura to the greater curve at the junction of the epiploics; this ensures an adequate blood supply to the stomach remnant.

Reconstruction can be completed by an esophagogastrostomy. Matthews and colleagues[10] described an effective and simple method to perform this type of anastomosis using a circular end-to-end anastomotic (EEA) stapler. The technique uses a flip-top 25-mm EEA stapler. A suture is passed between the top of the flipped anvil and the small hole in the tip of the anvil's post and tied; this secures the top into the flipped position. The distal end of a 16-French orogastric tube is transected proximal to its air port, and the anvil of the EEA stapler is then fit snugly into the lumen of the cut end of the orogastric tube (**Fig. 10**). A 2-0 silk stitch is used to secure the anvil in the distal end of the orogastric tube. Covidien Surgical (Mansfield, Massachusetts) now manufactures an already-modified circular EEA product in 21 and 25 mm diameters (DST Series EEA OrVil Devices) for this specific application, obviating the need for modification as originally described by Matthews and colleagues.[10]

The orogastric tube and anvil are coated with a sterile water-soluble lubricant, and the proximal portion of the orogastric tube is passed into the oropharynx and down the

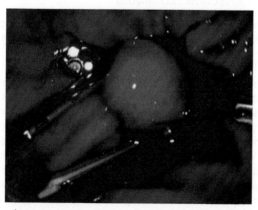

Fig. 9. Percutaneous, laparoscopic, intragastric stapled resection of submucosal tumor.

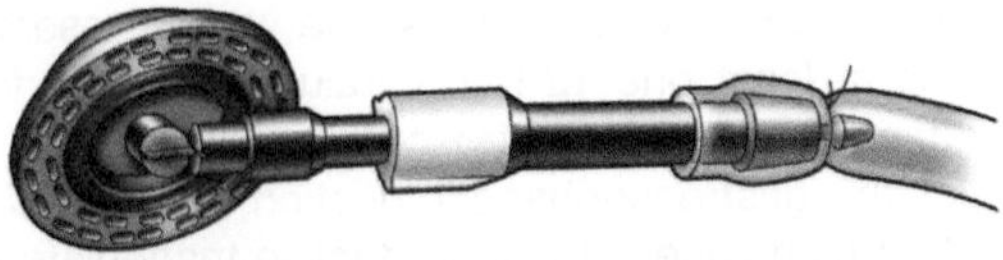

Fig. 10. Circular stapler anvil fashioned onto the proximal end of an orogastric tube. (*Courtesy of* B. Todd Heniford, MD, Carolinas Medical Center, Charlotte, NC.)

esophagus. A small enterotomy is made at the end of the esophagus, and the tube is gently pulled into the abdomen and out one of the trocar sites. The anvil is guided through the oropharynx under direct vision with a laryngoscope. When the anvil tip emerges from the esophagotomy, the sutures holding the anvil in the orogastric tube are cut, and the tube is split lengthwise over the anvil using the ultrasonic shears. This instrument quickly cuts through the plastic, allowing the orogastric tube to be pulled free and out of the abdomen. The EEA stapler is placed through an enlarged port site and advanced into a gastrotomy created in the gastric remnant. The spike of the EEA is advanced through the apex of the gastric remnant, and the anvil post and the stapler are united and fired. The gastrotomy is then closed with a GIA stapler or sewn intracorporeally, and a pyloromyotomy or pyloroplasty is performed.

Tumors of the Prepyloric Region

Tumors of the pyloric region are also amenable to laparoscopic resection. Intraluminal submucosal tumors of the pylorus are more difficult to resect than extraluminal tumors. Smaller tumors of the prepyloric region may be resected via a transgastric approach. A gastrotomy is made 6 cm proximal to the pylorus so that the pyloric muscle is not disrupted. The tumor is localized and 2 stay sutures are placed into the normal gastric tissue on either side of the tumor. The tumor is elevated through the gastrotomy and enucleated with hook cautery or resected with an endoscopic GIA stapler, taking care not to injure the pylorus. The initial gastrotomy is closed with sutures or a stapling device as previously described.

Large tumors of the prepyloric region can be treated in 1 of 2 ways. The first technique is an excision of the tumor with surrounding normal tissue using ultrasonic shears as previously described. A second technique is a formal antrectomy and Billroth II loop gastrojejunostomy, which is described in the following section.

FORMAL ANATOMIC RESECTION TECHNIQUES

Formal gastric resections are typically reserved for cases of refractory ulcer disease, reoperation for postgastrectomy syndromes, and select cases of malignancy.

Partial Gastrectomy

A partial gastric resection may range from an esophagogastrectomy procedure to antrectomy, subtotal, and near-total gastrectomy. In any of these procedures, the principles of gastric resection remain the same: resect only the necessary amount of gastric tissue and ensure an adequate blood supply to the remaining stomach.

Trocar positioning for formal anatomic gastric resection should be approximately 5 cm lower than that of the typical laparoscopic fundoplication trocar configuration. The author also adds an additional trocar to the right abdomen for the camera, and the previous camera port can be used for manipulation of the small bowel (**Fig. 11**).

The first step for any partial gastrectomy should be the division of the duodenum distal to the pylorus. The author begins by dividing the short gastric branches from

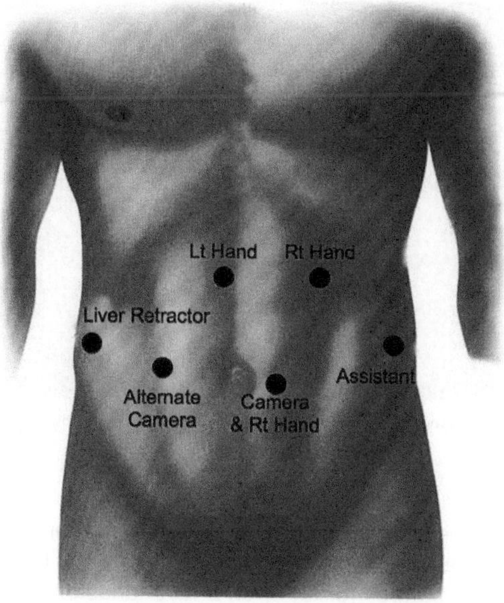

Fig. 11. Trocar configuration for formal anatomic gastric resections.

the gastroepiploic arteries along the lower greater curvature toward the patients' right side. The duodenum is then transected 1 cm distal to the pylorus (**Fig. 12**). The posterior aspect of the stomach is then mobilized and the division of the stomach can begin either along the lesser curvature or the greater curvature. To ensure complete antrectomy, the line of division runs from the incisura to the greater curvature at a point where the gastroepiploic vessel becomes indistinguishable from the stomach (**Fig. 13**).

Although a Billroth I gastroduodenostomy anastomosis can be performed laparoscopically, the author's preferred reconstruction technique is either a Billroth II loop or a roux en Y gastrojejunostomy. For a loop gastrojejunostomy, the ligament of Treitz is identified and a loop of jejunum that reaches easily into the upper abdomen is brought up toward the gastric pouch. The author prefers an antecolic gastrojejunostomy for its ease of construction. For increased mobility of the loop into the upper abdomen, the

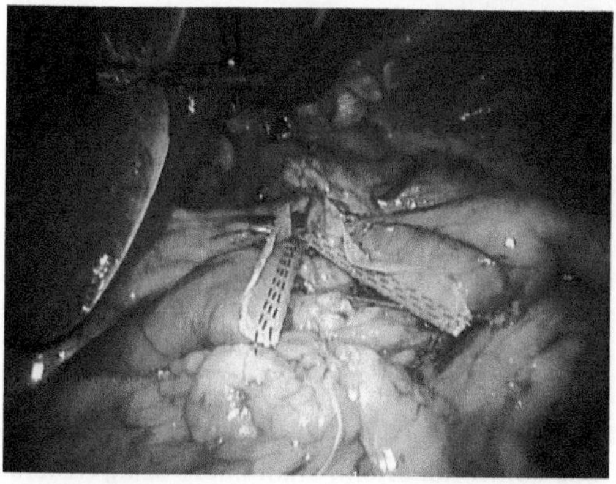

Fig. 12. Stapled transection of the duodenum as the initial step in laparoscopic antrectomy.

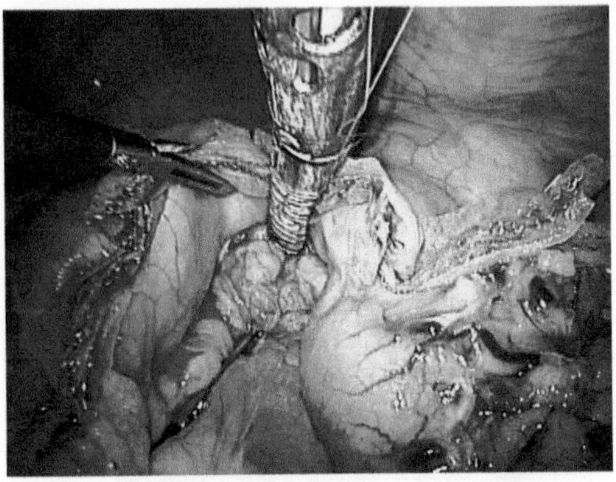

Fig. 13. Stapled transection of the stomach during antrectomy proceeding toward the greater curvature.

greater omentum may be split vertically with ultrasonic shears. To aid in the stapled anastomosis, stay sutures are placed from the jejunal loop to the gastric pouch much like the posterior row of sutures for an open 2-layer anastomosis. Utilizing an endoscopic GIA stapler with a 45-mm, blue, 3.5-mm staple height cartridge, the side-to-side gastrojejunostomy is created (**Fig. 14**). To aid in the stapled closure of the common enterotomy, stay sutures are placed to approximate the edges together (**Fig. 15**).

Alternatively, a roux en Y gastrojejunostomy reconstruction may be performed. The ligament of Treitz is identified, and an appropriate site is chosen to transect the jejunum. A roux limb of at least 50 cm is created, and a side-to-side stapled jejunojejunostomy is created (**Fig. 16**). The proximal roux limb is brought into the upper abdomen, and a side-to-side gastrojejunostomy is created as previously described.

Total Gastrectomy

Total gastrectomy is rarely indicated other than for malignant disease. The reconstruction of intestinal continuity is one of the most difficult because it requires an esophagojejunostomy. Trocar configuration is as previously described, and the complete gastric resection is straightforward.

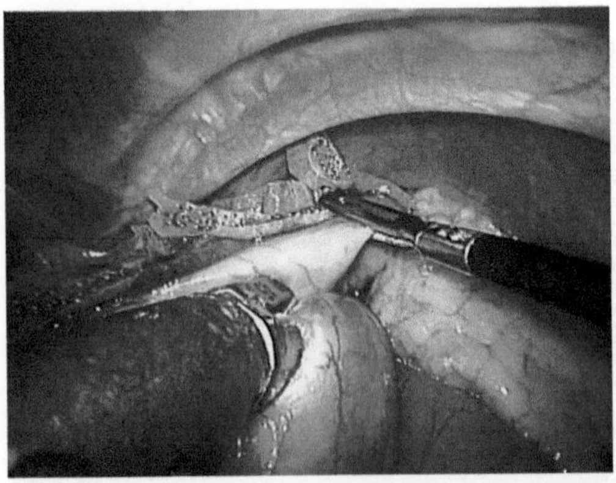

Fig. 14. Side-to-side loop gastrojejunostomy anastomosis being created with an endoscopic GIA stapler.

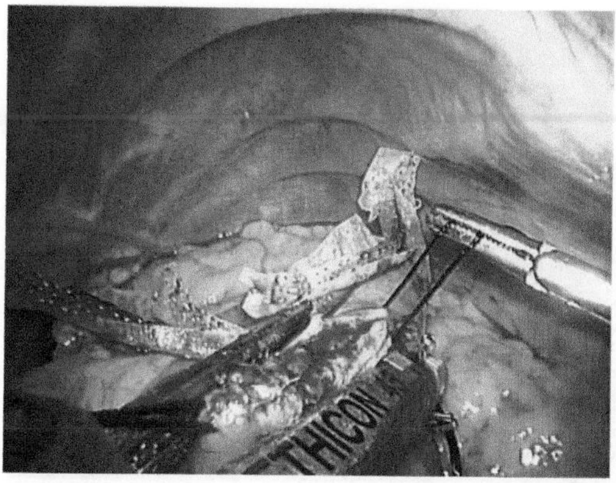

Fig. 15. Stapled closure of the common enterotomy after creation of the side-to-side loop gastrojejunostomy anastomosis.

The duodenum is divided first, and the lesser curvature is mobilized toward the right crus. A minimal crural dissection allows for the mobilization of esophageal length into the abdominal cavity. Following the esophageal mobilization, the greater curvature is mobilized and separated from the spleen. Utilizing an endoscopic GIA stapler with a 45-mm, blue, 3.5-mm staple height cartridge, the esophagus is transected at the gastroesophageal junction. To prevent retraction into the mediastinum after transection, lateral stay sutures can be placed into the esophagus to aid with intraabdominal retraction.

The roux en Y esophagojejunostomy is created using the orogastric tube circular stapler anvil technique previously described. After creation of the roux limb, the EEA stapler anvil, attached to an orogastric tube, is advanced transorally, and the tube with the attached anvil is delivered through an end esophagotomy. The tube is then disconnected from the anvil. The staple line of the proximal roux limb is opened with ultrasonic shears and the circular EEA stapler, passed through an enlarged trocar skin incision in the left lateral abdomen, and is advanced into the open roux end. The spike is advanced through the antimesenteric border of the roux limb and the limb is taken into the upper abdomen where the spike is united with the transesophageal anvil,

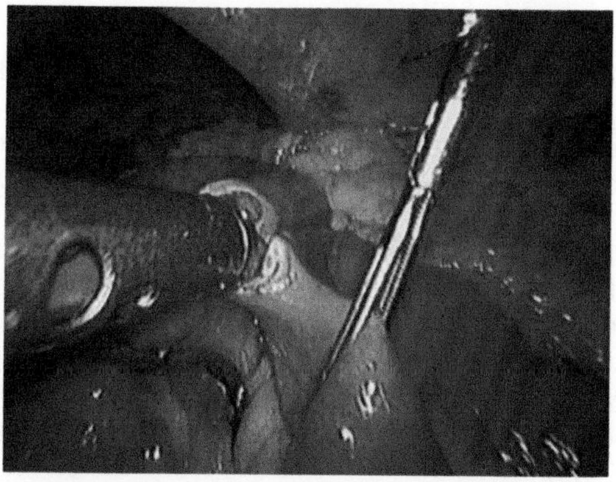

Fig. 16. Side-to-side stapled jejunojejunostomy being created.

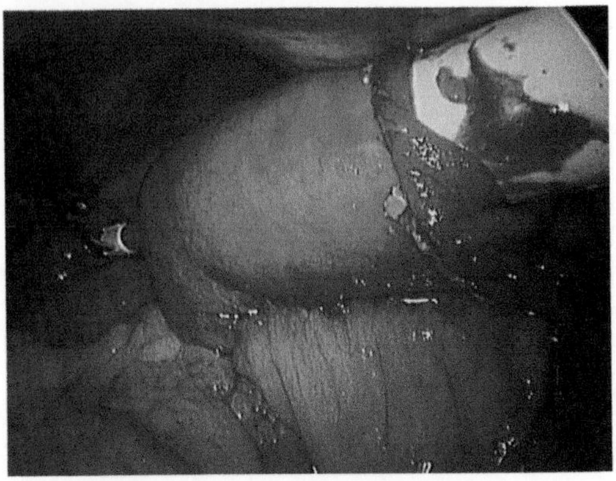

Fig. 17. End-to-side esophagojejunostomy anastomosis being created with circular EEA stapler advanced through the proximal end of the roux limb.

and a circular anastomosis is created (**Fig. 17**). Later, the open end of the roux limb is staple transected with an endoscopic GIA stapler.

SUMMARY

Laparoscopic techniques for gastric resection are bountiful and require knowledge of the anatomy; resourcefulness; flexible endoscopic skills; and a good understanding of modern trocars, energy sources, and endoscopic staplers. As long as the basic principles of open surgery are adhered to when performing laparoscopy, patients will benefit from these less-invasive approaches to benign and malignant diseases of the stomach.

ACKNOWLEDGMENTS

The author would like to thank Anne Olson, the artist who created the illustrations for this article, and B. Todd Heniford, MD, Chief, Division of Gastrointestinal and Minimally Invasive Surgery of the Carolinas Medical Center (Charlotte, NC), who granted permission for the use of these illustrations.

REFERENCES

1. Silas AM, Kruskal JB, Kane RA. Intraoperative ultrasound. Radiol Clin North Am 2001;39:429.
2. Kane RA. Laparoscopic ultrasound. In: Kane RA, editor. Intraoperative, laparoscopic, and endoluminal ultrasound. Philadelphia: Churchill Livingstone; 1999. p. 90.
3. Jakimowicz J, Stultiens G. Ultrasound techniques in minimal-access surgery. In: Greene F, Heniford B, editors. Minimally invasive cancer management. 1st edition. New York: Springer-Verlag; 2001. p. 75.
4. Schauer PR, Ikramuddin S, Gourash W, et al. Outcomes after laparoscopic Roux-en-Y gastric bypass for morbid obesity. Ann Surg 2000;232:515.
5. Dapri G, Cadiere GB, Himpens J. Reinforcing the staple line during laparoscopic sleeve gastrectomy: prospective randomized clinical study comparing three different techniques. Obes Surg 2010;20:462.

6. Jones WB, Myers KM, Traxler LB, et al. Clinical results using bioabsorbable staple line reinforcement for circular staplers. Am Surg 2008;74:462.
7. Ohashi S. Laparoscopic intraluminal (intragastric) surgery for early gastric cancer. A new concept in laparoscopic surgery. Surg Endosc 1995;9:169.
8. Heniford BT, Arca MJ, Walsh RM. The mini-laparoscopic intragastric resection of a gastroesophageal stromal tumor: a novel approach. Surg Laparosc Endosc Percutan Tech 2000;10:82.
9. Demetri GD, Benjamin RS, Blanke CD, et al. NCCN Task Force report: management of patients with gastrointestinal stromal tumor (GIST)–update of the NCCN clinical practice guidelines. J Natl Compr Canc Netw 2007;5(Suppl 2):S1.
10. Matthews BD, Sing RF, DeLegge MH, et al. Initial results with a stapled gastrojejunostomy for the laparoscopic isolated roux-en-Y gastric bypass. Am J Surg 2000;179:476.

Postgastrectomy Syndromes

John S. Bolton, MD[a,b,*], W. Charles Conway II, MD[a]

KEYWORDS

• Postgastrectomy syndromes • Diagnosis • Management

The first postgastrectomy syndrome was noted not long after the first gastrectomy was performed: Billroth[1] reported a case of epigastric pain associated with bilious vomiting as a sequel of gastric surgery in 1885. Several classic treatises exist on the subject; we cannot improve on them and merely provide a few references for the interested reader.[1–3]

However, the indications for gastric resection have changed dramatically over the past 4 decades, and the overall incidence of gastric resection has decreased. The most marked reduction in the frequency of gastric resection has occurred among patients with peptic ulcer disease. For example, in Olmstead County, Minnesota, the incidence of elective operations on previously unoperated patients declined 8-fold during the 30-year study period between 1956 and 1985[4] and undoubtedly has declined even further since. One population-based study concluded that elective surgery for ulcer disease had "virtually disappeared by 1992–1996."[5] Whereas emergency operations for bleeding and perforation are still encountered, acid-reducing procedures are being performed less frequently in these situations in favor of a damage control approach.[6] Even for gastric cancer, resection rates decreased approximately 20% from 1988 to 2000 in the United States.[7] An estimated 21,000 new cases of stomach cancer occurred in the United States in 2010,[8] so that the number of cases of gastric resection for cancer is probably less than 15,000 per year in the United States. The virtual disappearance of elective surgery for peptic ulcer has also changed the demographic profile of the postgastrectomy patient: patients who have gastric cancer tend to be older and there is only a slight male preponderance. These significant changes in the gastric surgery population make it worthwhile to revisit postgastrectomy syndromes.

The frequency with which postgastrectomy symptoms/syndromes are found can depend on how hard they are looked for. Loffeld,[9] in a survey of 124 postgastrectomy

The authors have no financial interests to disclose.

[a] Department of Surgery Ochsner Clinic Foundation, 1514 Jefferson Highway, New Orleans, LA 70121, USA

[b] The University of Queensland School of Medicine-Ochsner Clinical School, USA

* Corresponding author.

E-mail address: JBOLTON@ochsner.org

Surg Clin N Am 91 (2011) 1105–1122

doi:10.1016/j.suc.2011.07.001

surgical.theclinics.com

0039-6109/11/$ – see front matter © 2011 Elsevier Inc. All rights reserved.

patients, most of whom had undergone surgery more than 15 years earlier, found that 75% suffered from upper abdominal symptoms, and 1 or more symptoms that indicate dumping were found in 70% of patients who had undergone Billroth-II (B-II) reconstruction. However, the lack of age-matched and sex-matched controls in this study may have overstated the frequency of symptoms caused by the surgical procedure. Mine and colleagues[10] conducted a large survey of 1153 patients after gastrectomy for cancer and found that 67% reported early dumping and 38% late dumping. By contrast, Pedrazzani and colleagues[11] surveyed 195 patients who underwent subtotal gastrectomy and B-II reconstruction for gastric adenocarcinoma for up to 5 years postoperatively, and concluded that "the incidence of late complications was low and the majority of them recovered within one year after surgery." Our personal experience tends to corroborate that most patients have a good functional result after gastric resection for cancer, provided that the cancer is cured. This article focuses on the small proportion of patients with severe, debilitating symptoms; these symptoms can challenge the acumen of the surgeon who is providing the patient's long-term follow-up and care.

This article does not attempt to deal with the sequelae of bariatric surgery, which has become the most common indication for elective gastric surgery with an estimated 71,190 patients having laparoscopic gastric bypass in the United States in 2006.[12]

NUTRITIONAL AND METABOLIC SEQUELAE

Virtually all patients who submit to subtotal or total gastrectomy experience significant weight loss within the first several months postoperatively. On average, the amount of weight lost is approximately 10% of preoperative weight. Body weight usually stabilizes by 3 months postoperatively, in the absence of superimposed clinical problems. Body composition studies performed at 6 and 12 months postoperatively reveal that the weight loss is comprised entirely of body fat and that lean body cell mass is unchanged.[13] If this loss of body fat were the only consequence of gastric resection, one would probably ascribe it as a benefit.

The incidence of significant bone disorders after gastrectomy is considerable. Zittel and colleagues[14] found that 55% of 60 gastrectomized patients had vertebral fractures or osteopenia when studied 5 to 20 years after gastrectomy. The risk of having a vertebral deformity was increased 6-fold after gastrectomy compared with age-matched and sex-matched controls. Approximately half of the patients in this study had undergone gastrectomy for peptic ulcer disease and the other half for carcinoma, and the magnitude of bone disorder was similar for both groups. Forty of the study patients had undergone distal subtotal gastrectomy, with 20 Billroth-I (B-I) and 20 B-II reconstructions, and the prevalence of bone abnormality was similar between them. Twenty patients in this study had undergone total gastrectomy, and the prevalence of postgastrectomy bone disease was greatest in this group.[14] In a population-based study of patients who underwent surgery for peptic ulcer in Rochester, Minnesota between 1956 and 1985, the risk of distal radial, proximal femur, and vertebral fracture was increased between 2.2-fold and 4.7-fold at a median follow-up of 14.8 years.[15] The most likely explanation for postgastrectomy bone disorder seems to be decreased calcium absorption caused by bypass of upper small bowel absorptive area in patients reconstructed by B-II and Roux-Y techniques and caused by decreased dissolution and ionization of calcium salts in an acid-free environment after gastrectomy.[16] Milk intolerance, maldigestion caused by pancreatic insufficiency or pancreaticocibal asynchrony, malabsorption caused by rapid food transit, or steatorrhea leading to the formation of insoluble calcium soaps are other possible mechanisms.[14] Several studies report that the accelerated bone density loss after gastrectomy occurs early (within the first 2–3 years postoperatively), suggesting that therapeutic intervention needs to be started soon after surgery.[17,18] In animal models, feeding soluble fiber or nondigestible disaccharides after total gastrectomy improved calcium absorption and protected against osteopenia.[19,20] Postgastrectomy effects on vitamin D metabolism and parathyroid hormone secretion have not been well characterized.

Severe copper deficiency presenting as a syndrome of ataxia, myelopathy, and peripheral neuropathy, clinically mimicking vitamin B_{12} deficiency, has been reported in patients undergoing prior gastrectomy.[21,22] Copper is absorbed primarily in the duodenum.

Anemia is common among patients undergoing prior gastrectomy. Ingested iron is absorbed primarily in the duodenum, which is bypassed with either B-II or Roux-Y reconstruction after gastric resection. Also, ingested iron must be reduced by the acid environment of the stomach to be efficiently absorbed. Ingested vitamin B_{12} requires intrinsic factor, produced by the proximal stomach, to be absorbed. In 1 study, among 72 patients evaluated for anemia after prior gastrectomy 94% had iron deficiency anemia and 79% had vitamin B_{12} deficiency; combinations of the 2 were present in most patients. By contrast, folate deficiency was uncommon, occurring in only 4% of the patients with anemia.[23] In an experimental model, ingestion of a nondigestible disaccharide prevented gastrectomy-induced iron malabsorption and anemia, possibly by cecal fermentation of the disaccharide,[24] but this therapy has not been applied in human studies. Iron deficiency anemia in a postgastrectomy patient should not be presumed to be caused by the postgastrectomy state without first ruling out other clinically significant disease in the upper and lower gastrointestinal tract by endoscopy.[25]

DUMPING SYNDROME

The dumping syndrome is caused by rapid gastric emptying as a result of loss of pyloric regulation of gastric emptying and, possibly, impaired accommodation of the proximal gastric remnant.[26] The rapid emptying of liquid-phase simple sugars presents the small bowel with a large, nonphysiologic, hyperosmolar solute load. Symptoms of early dumping include crampy abdominal pain and diarrhea within 30 minutes after oral intake, associated with weakness, light-headedness, and rapid heart rate. These symptoms are mediated by local peristaltic responses in the gastrointestinal tract, plasma volume changes, gut hormones (including insulin and glucagonlike peptide), and humoral factors including norepinephrine.[27,28] Objective criteria for diagnosis and correlation with a provocative test using an oral challenge with 50 g of glucose have been developed.[29] Late dumping occurs approximately 2 hours after meals, and the symptoms are those of hypoglycemia. The mechanism probably involves a reactive hypoglycemia brought on by the rapid and high initial glucose load presented to and absorbed by the small intestine, resulting in an inappropriately high insulin response, leading to hypoglycemia. Both early and late dumping may also be seen after surgical procedures that only incidentally remove the distal stomach or ablate the pylorus, such as the classic Whipple procedure or esophagogastrectomy for esophageal cancer in which pyloromyotomy or pyloroplasty is added.

In a retrospective study of 310 patients undergoing distal subtotal gastrectomy with B-II reconstruction for gastric cancer, Pedrazzani and colleagues[11] noted that the dumping syndrome was uncommon and tended to resolve with time, being present in only 5% of patients 2 years after surgery. However, for the small number of patients affected, symptoms can be severe, life-altering, and debilitating.[27]

Mine and colleagues,[10] in a survey of 1153 patients after gastrectomy for gastric cancer, found on multivariate analysis that early dumping syndrome was significantly less likely to occur in older patients, patients undergoing pylorus-preserving gastrectomy, and patients having Roux-Y reconstruction after distal gastrectomy. Late dumping syndrome was significantly more frequent among patients who had early dumping syndrome or were female. Nunobe and colleagues[30] compared the results of B-I and Roux-Y reconstruction in 385 patients undergoing subtotal distal gastrectomy for early gastric cancer. In a gastrointestinal quality-of-life survey carried out 5 years after surgery, no significant differences were found between the Roux-Y and B-I groups with respect to symptoms of early or late postprandial dumping. This finding is not surprising because dumping is a result of resection of the pylorus and is unaffected by the type of reconstruction.

Initial therapy consists of dietary evaluation and counseling. Daily intake should be divided into at least 6 meals. Liquids should be avoided with meals. Diets should be high in protein and fat, and simple sugars should be avoided. Vasomotor symptoms can often be ameliorated if the patient lies down for 30 minutes after meals.

For patients with severe postgastrectomy dumping symptoms refractory to diet therapy, the somatostatin analogue octreotide is the pharmacologic therapy of choice. It acts through its inhibitory effects on insulin and gut hormone release, a delay of intestinal transit time, and inhibition of food-induced circulatory changes. A review of 7 small randomized controlled trials (RCTs) of short-acting octreotide for the treatment of severe dumping syndrome found evidence of significant clinical benefit in all studies and recommended the use of octreotide for severe or refractory dumping syndrome.[31] In a comparative study of octreotide taken 3 times a day versus monthly long-acting repeatable octreotide in 30 patients with dumping syndrome unresponsive to dietary intervention, the formulations were equally effective in blunting objective measures of the dumping syndrome, but the long-acting preparation scored significantly better on quality-of-life measures.[32] These findings were confirmed by a crossover study among 12 patients reported by Penning and colleagues.[33] However, octreotide therapy for dumping was found to lose efficacy over time: in a long-term study by Didden and colleagues,[34] 50% of patients with initial excellent relief of symptoms discontinued therapy because of side effects or loss of efficacy, and Vecht and colleagues[35] found that long-term use is frequently limited by side effects, chiefly diarrhea and steatorrhea. Acarbose, 50 mg 3 times per day, can be used for the prevention of late dumping.[36,37] Acarbose is a competitive inhibitor of α-glycoside hydrolase and delays carbohydrate digestion and absorption.

A surgical approach to the primary prevention of the dumping syndrome (the preservation of an intact pylorus in patients with early gastric cancer of the midbody of the stomach [segmental gastrectomy]) has been extensively evaluated in Japan and has been shown to significantly decrease the incidence of postoperative dumping.[38–41] The preservation of an intact anteropyloric grinding mechanism with a reduction of the capacitance function of the proximal stomach after resection can serve to promote esophageal reflux. This is the argument against extensive proximal gastrectomy with pyloric preservation. Another surgical approach to treat dumping that has been described and is included for completeness is the use of a reversed 10-cm jejunal segment to slow the transit of intestinal contents.[42,43] The twisting of a segment of bowel on its mesentery violates the tenets of gastrointestinal surgery and we do not favor it.

However, caution should be exercised when preserving the pylorus after proximal gastrectomy with jejunal interposition: Nakane and colleagues[44] found a significantly higher incidence of delayed gastric emptying, reflux gastritis, and bile regurgitation, and suboptimal weight maintenance 1 year postoperatively among patients in whom pyloroplasty was omitted during proximal gastrectomy with jejunal interposition. These problems might be overcome by preserving vagal innervations to the pylorus.[45]

AFFERENT LOOP SYNDROME

This entity is mentioned mostly out of historical interest; we have not seen a case for many years. The virtual disappearance of this postgastrectomy syndrome is because of the dramatic decrease in the frequency with which partial gastrectomy and B-II reconstructions are performed for peptic ulcer disease. Diagnosis is made almost entirely based on the patient's history of repetitive episodes of postprandial right upper abdominal colicky pain building to a crescendo, culminating in almost projectile bilious vomiting with simultaneous relief of pain. In a patient with this history, the diagnosis may be corroborated by a computed tomography scan showing chronic dilation of the duodenum, or by right upper quadrant ultrasound after a provocative meal to show the acute distension of the afferent limb. When afferent loop syndrome is diagnosed, reoperation is required to either revise the B-II anastomosis or to convert to a Roux-Y reconstruction. Another possible solution to afferent loop syndrome is an afferent to efferent loop bypass. This bypass procedure, originally described by Braun,[46] is particularly useful when dissection of the original gastrojejunal anastomosis is not required or technically difficult.

DELAYED GASTRIC EMPTYING

Severe, prolonged delayed gastric emptying that prevents oral alimentation is rare after gastric resection for cancer. However, food retention in the gastric remnant after distal subtotal gastrectomy for cancer is commonly seen at postoperative endoscopy. Jung and colleagues[47] found food retention at endoscopy in 21% of patients at 24 months postoperatively after an overnight fast. The incidence of food retention was higher after B-I than after B-II reconstruction. Kubo and colleagues[48] reported a similar incidence of food retention after distal subtotal gastrectomy for gastric cancer and found that food retention was more frequent after B-I than after Roux-Y reconstruction. However, none of the patients in either of these studies had clinically significant delayed gastric emptying, and no association was found between food retention and symptoms or body weight change. The medical management and strategies to restore gastric electrical stimulation to treat delayed gastric emptying are thoroughly covered elsewhere in this issue and are not included in this section. When delayed gastric emptying symptoms affect a patient's quality of life and medical management or pacing fails, reducing or eliminating the remnant stomach is the only option. Speicher and colleagues[49] reported a series of 44 patients over a 20-year period who required completion gastrectomy for chronic gastric atony after prior gastric surgery. The indication for the initial gastric operation was peptic ulcer disease in 75%, morbid obesity in 11%, gastroesophageal reflux disease in 9%, and bile reflux in 5%.

ROUX STASIS

Roux stasis, or Roux limb syndrome, is characterized by abdominal pain, nausea, vomiting, and postprandial bloating. Although some investigators report up to a 30% incidence, others have not found this syndrome to be nearly as clinically relevant.[50]

Although debating this entity may be academic, the physiologic changes possibly causing it are worthy of discussion.

Pacesetter potentials are cyclical electrical changes in the small bowel.[51] These potentials are fastest in the duodenal pacemaker and spread distally to the terminal ileum, generating action potentials that induce muscle contraction along the way. When the jejunum is transected, the frequency of pacesetter potentials in the distal bowel decreases and ectopic pacemakers appear that drive the potentials retrograde, toward the stomach.[52] Canine studies have revealed reduced transit of liquids through the segment of bowel with orally moving pacesetter potentials, and provide a physiologic explanation for the Roux stasis syndrome.[52] However, correlation of symptoms in human subjects has not been so definitive. Miedema and colleagues[53] found that although transit was uniformly slowed in the Roux limb, there was not a transit difference between asymptomatic patients and those with stasis symptoms.

Bile Reflux Gastritis

This entity seems to be less common now than it was in the past. The most likely explanation for this situation is that Roux-Y reconstruction after distal subtotal gastrectomy for cancer has been preferred by most surgeons in the United States for many years, and cancer resections have become the most common indication for gastrectomy with the precipitous decline in surgery for peptic ulcer disease. A previously cited study comparing B-I and Roux-Y reconstructions 5 years after distal subtotal gastrectomy for cancer showed a significantly lower incidence of gastritis on endoscopy and fewer symptoms of epigastric discomfort after Roux-Y compared with B-I.[30] A similar type of comparative retrospective study of Roux-Y, B-I, and B-II anatomy using a quality-of-life survey and quantitative measurement of bile reflux using the Bilitec (Synectics Medical AB, Stockholm, Sweden) probe showed significantly fewer symptoms and less bile reflux in the Roux-Y group.[54] Better outcomes with Roux-Y than with B-II were also seen in a study by Kronert and colleagues[55] using the Bilitec probe and a symptom survey in a group of patients after partial gastrectomy for benign peptic ulcer disease. Another recent study compared Roux versus B-I versus B-II patients 14 days after surgery for gastric cancer with the Bilitec probe and found bile reflux to be significantly less with Roux-Y reconstruction (B-II reconstruction had the highest incidence of bile reflux, noted in 70% of patients).[56] Endoscopy 3 months postoperatively showed significantly less reflux gastritis in Roux-Y patients, although symptom surveys were not significantly different between the 3 groups. Remnant gastritis was not affected by *Helicobacter pylori* status in this study.

Csendes and colleagues[57] reported the status after an average of 15.5 years of 75 patients randomized to Roux-Y versus B-II reconstruction after vagotomy and distal gastrectomy for duodenal ulcer disease. Roux-Y patients had fewer symptoms, better Visick scores, and an absence of chronic gastritis on endoscopy (vs an 80% incidence of chronic gastritis in the B-II group), despite the fact that *H pylori* was present in a similar proportion of patients. In a study (nonrandomized) by Fukuhara and colleagues[58] comparing Roux-Y versus B-I versus B-II patients 3 months after distal gastrectomy for cancer, interleukin 8 levels in gastric mucosa (on endoscopic biopsy specimens) were significantly lower in Roux patients both in the absence and the presence of active *H pylori* infection. They concluded that Roux Y reconstruction is better able to prevent remnant gastritis.

Although bile reflux and gastritis are more common after B-I and B-II reconstruction than after Roux-Y, debilitating symptoms are infrequent. For the few patients with severe bile reflux gastritis after partial or subtotal distal gastrectomy with B-I or B-II reconstruction, the best solution is to reoperate and convert to Roux-Y anatomy.

Reflux Esophagitis

Available evidence suggests that Roux-Y reconstruction results in a lower incidence of reflux esophagitis compared with B-I or B-II reconstruction. One study relates this to the preservation of a narrow angle of His with Roux-Y.[59] Nunobe and colleagues[30] showed a significantly lower incidence of heartburn symptoms and grade B or worse esophagitis in Roux-Y patients than in B-I patients after distal subtotal gastrectomy for early gastric cancer. Csendes and colleagues[57] found that Roux-Y patients had significantly less esophagitis on endoscopy and less Barrett metaplasia, compared with B-II patients, in a study of 75 patients randomized to Roux-Y versus B-I reconstruction after vagotomy and distal gastrectomy for duodenal ulcer disease studied 15.5 years after operation.

Cholelithiasis, Biliary Colic, and Cholecystitis

In a series of 463 patients with a normal gallbladder who underwent gastrectomy for gastric cancer and survived the operation, 85 of the 281 patients who underwent radical gastrectomy and 9 of the 182 patients who underwent simple gastrectomy developed gallstones ($P<.001$).[60] The mean interval between gastrectomy and gallstone formation was shorter in the radical gastrectomy patients (31.4 ± 20.9 months) than in the simple gastrectomy patients (48.0 ± 12.8 months) ($P<.05$). The investigators recommend prophylactic cholecystectomy on patients with a normal gallbladder having radical gastrectomy. Nunobe and colleagues[30] found a significantly higher incidence of postoperative gallstone formation in the Roux-Y group (28%) than in the B-I group (15%) 5 years after distal subtotal gastrectomy for early gastric cancer. The increased risk of gallstone formation is related to loss of vagal innervation of the gallbladder with decreased gallbladder motility after radical gastrectomy, and a result of loss of cholecystokinin release from the duodenum with bypass of the duodenum when Roux-Y reconstruction is performed.

Recurrent/Anastomotic Ulceration

Recurrent ulceration after peptic ulcer surgery most commonly results from incomplete vagotomy and nonsteroidal antiinflammatory drug use.[61] The most common sites for recurrence include peripyloric, duodenal, and peristomal areas. The role of *H pylori* is less clear than in the cases of initial peptic ulcer.[62] Treatment consists of proton pump inhibitors and discontinuing ulcerogenic medications. When this treatment fails, and incomplete vagotomy is diagnosed, transthoracic truncal vagotomy is recommended.[63]

Less common causes include hypersecretory states (Zollinger-Ellison syndrome) and retained antrum. In cases of retained antrum, there is residual antral tissue within the duodenal stump after gastric resection with B-II anastomosis. The G cells are continuously bathed in alkaline duodenal fluid, resulting in continuous secretion of gastrin, causing sustained intense stimulation of acid production by parietal cells in the proximal stomach remnant. The exposure of the unprotected jejunum to this high acid level results in what is termed a marginal ulcer (**Fig. 1**). Diagnosis can be made with a sodium 99m technetium scan, and reexcision is curative.

Gastric Remnant Carcinoma

The risk of cancer in the stomach remnant after partial gastrectomy has been debated for many years.[64–66] However, early studies suffered from a heterogeneous patient mix, including patients with peptic ulcer disease and gastric cancer, and from not ensuring patients with gastric ulcers did not have a missed gastric cancer. More

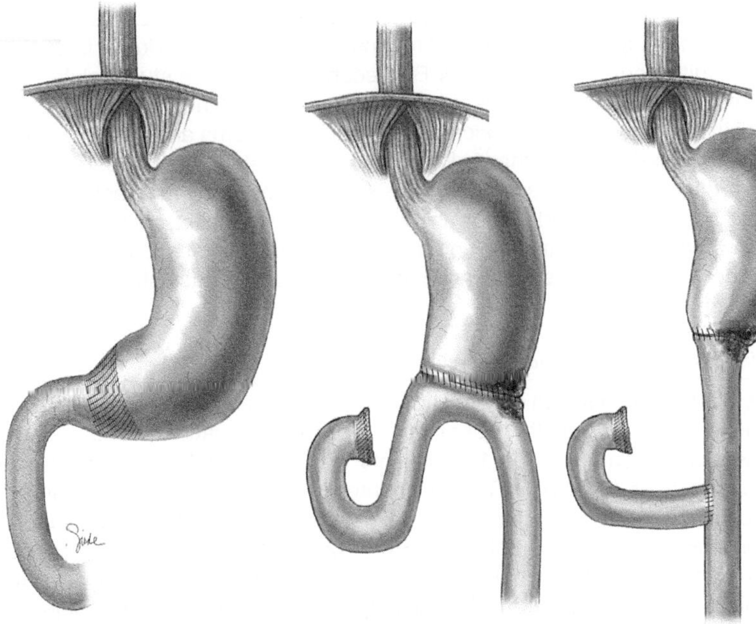

Fig. 1. Pathophysiology of retained antrum syndrome: incompletely resected antrum during distal gastrectomy with B-II or Roux-Y reconstruction results in intense gastrin secretion by the remaining antrum, which is constantly bathed in the alkaline environment of the adjoined duodenum.

recently, larger studies, limited to patients with clearly benign disease, incorporating selection criteria to minimize pathologic error, have been reported, although without absolute consensus. In a review of 1000 patients who had gastric resection with B-II reconstruction for duodenal ulcer, Fischer and colleagues[67] noted only 13 cases of remnant carcinoma, not different from the general population using the life table method. Viste and colleagues[68] noted remnant carcinoma in 87 of 3470 (2.5%) postgastrectomy patients with initially benign disease, with an observed/expected ratio of 2.1 (P<.001). Risk was not increased in the first 5 to 10 years after surgery, but after 40 to 45 years it was 7.3-fold higher than the expected value for the population. In 1988, 2 published cancer registry-based studies only added to the controversy, with differing conclusions.[69,70] As had been noted by previous investigators, the Swedish study[70] revealed an increased remnant cancer risk in patients with a B-II reconstruction compared with those with a B-I and in patients undergoing gastrectomy for gastric ulcer compared with those with other benign diseases. In 1993, a Veterans Affairs study[71] compared more than 7000 patients undergoing gastric resection for a benign disorder with a matched control group and noted an increased risk of remnant cancer (standardized rate ratio 1.9, confidence interval 1.3–2.4), especially in those with gastric ulcer.

Although absolute consensus may be lacking, physiologic changes related to gastrectomy could produce a procarcinogenic state. Miwa and colleagues[72] found duodenal reflux into the rat stomach induced adenocarcinoma. Ruddell and colleagues[73] reported an increase in gastric juice nitrite concentrations in hypochlorhydric subjects, and it is known that hypochlorhydria allows increased luminal bacteria that are able to convert nitrates to nitrites.[74] Nitrites are precursors of the known carcinogenic *N*-nitroso compounds, more commonly noted in the remnant after B-II reconstruction.[75] Furthermore, secondary bile acids, known to promote gastritis and metaplasia, constantly bathe the gastric stump anastomosis after B-II and may explain a recent report that remnant carcinomas after B-II are more likely at the intestinal anastomosis, whereas after B-I they are noted equally throughout the stomach.[76]

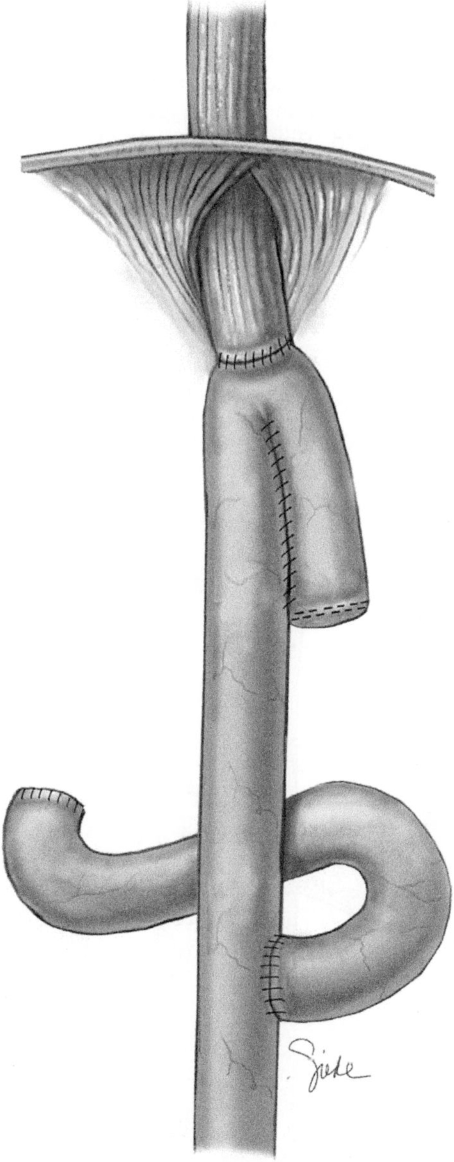

Fig. 2. Proximal pouch Roux-Y reconstruction.

Although many papers have been published on the risk of remnant carcinoma, perspective is needed. Caygill and colleagues[77] reviewed outcomes on more than 5000 patients undergoing gastric resection. Whereas 37 deaths resulted from remnant gastric cancer in patients living longer than 20 years, there were 991 deaths from lung cancer and nonneoplastic causes. With 80% of patients with peptic ulcers being smokers,[78] efforts at lifestyle modification rather than endoscopic screening of the gastric remnant may be more fruitful in improving the long-term outcome of the post-gastrectomy patient.

Does the Quality of Life After Gastrectomy Depend on the Type of Reconstruction?

A nonrandomized retrospective comparison of B-I, B-II, and Roux-Y 3 years after partial gastrectomy, including multiple end points (Visick grading, dumping score, afferent and efferent loop syndromes, bile reflux, regurgitation, overall quality of life) found significantly better outcomes with Roux-Y reconstruction.[79] A second retrospective comparison of B-I and Roux-Y reconstruction 5 years after distal

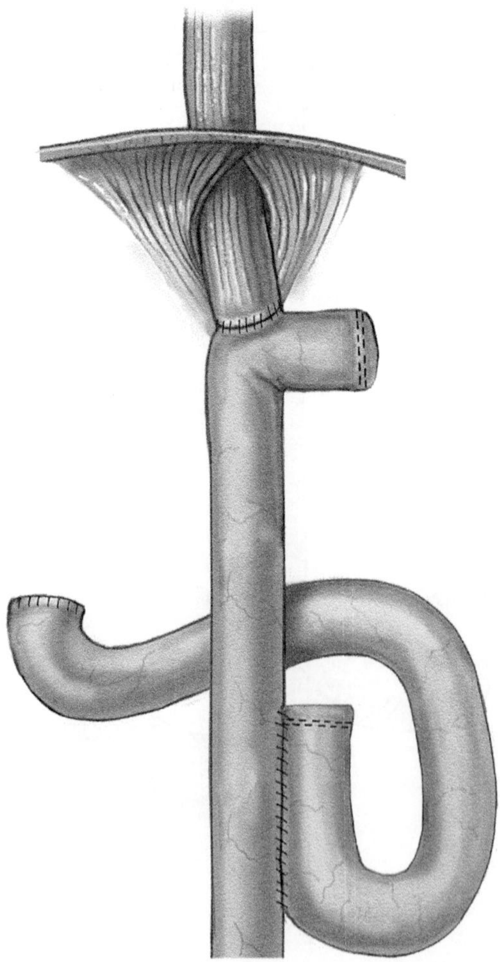

Fig. 3. Distal pouch Roux-Y reconstruction.

gastrectomy for early gastric cancer found that Roux-Y reconstruction was superior; however, the incidence of gallstone development was higher after Roux-Y.[30] In a randomized comparison of B-II and Roux-Y reconstruction after vagotomy and distal gastrectomy for duodenal ulcer, Roux-Y patients had significantly fewer postoperative symptoms and better Visick grading than did B-II patients ($P<.001$).[57] However, another small randomized comparison of Roux-Y versus B-I reconstruction after distal gastrectomy for gastric cancer found a significantly longer hospital stay in the Roux-Y group ($P<.05$) as a result of gastrojejunal stasis and no significant difference in postoperative nutritional status.[80]

After Total Gastrectomy, Does a Pouch Matter?

Construction of a jejunal pouch as a substitute for the stomach after total gastrectomy was first proposed by Hunt in 1952.[81] The technique has not been widely accepted, but multiple RCTs over the past 15 years have, for the most part, supported the use of a pouch.[13,82–91] These RCTs have been small in size and have used different techniques for pouch construction. The differences between the pouch and nonpouch groups have been modest. Examples of several techniques of pouch reconstruction are provided in **Figs. 2–4**. A recent meta-analysis encountered several methodologic difficulties but concluded that "a pouch reconstruction after total gastrectomy is clearly beneficial for patients with expected long-term survival."[92,93] The benefit was

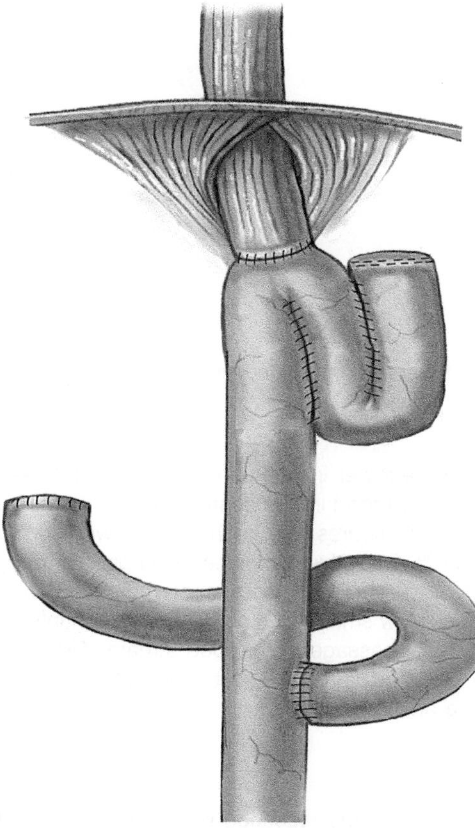

Fig. 4. S pouch Roux-Y reconstruction creating a larger reservoir.

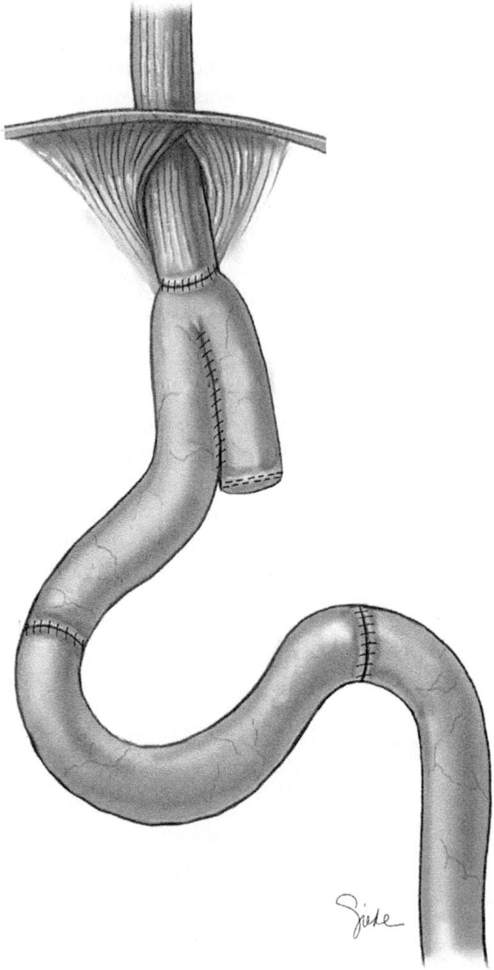

Fig. 5. Pouch interposition: note that duodenal continuity with the food stream is maintained.

most clearly evident in the lower incidence of dumping and heartburn reported by patients and higher reported food intake postoperatively. In particular, the Gastrointestinal Quality of Life Index scores for pouch patients were significantly better than for nonpouch patients.[90] Objective evidence of improved body weight was not reported in this meta-analysis. The findings apply only to Roux-Y pouch formation after total gastrectomy. A few small RCTs comparing pouch interposition reconstruction (maintaining duodenal passage of the food stream, **Fig. 5**) with Roux-Y pouch reconstruction have reported variable results; overall, the studies are not robust enough to permit meta-analysis.[85,88,94,95]

SUMMARY

The frequency with which gastric resection is performed in the United States has decreased significantly over the past 4 decades. As a direct result of this situation, the number of patients with severe postgastrectomy syndromes is probably decreasing. Gastric cancer resection is the most frequent indication for gastrectomy in the United States and worldwide. As long-term survival rates for patients who have resected gastric cancer improve, long-term quality of life is increasingly important; this is already true in East Asia, where 60% of gastric cancers are early and innovative new techniques are being used to avoid or minimize postgastrectomy symptoms. Most patients who have gastric cancer maintain healthy body weight and lean body mass postoperatively and have satisfactory gastrointestinal quality of life after gastric resection, but a small number (<5%) have persistent debilitating symptoms of a postgastrectomy syndrome. In this article, the major postgastrectomy syndromes are presented and their prevention and treatment discussed. After total gastrectomy for cancer, Roux-Y reconstruction is preferred. There is no evidence that the added operative time required to recreate the reservoir function of the stomach by pouch reconstruction is warranted. The incidence of gallstones after gastrectomy is significant.

REFERENCES

1. Ritchie WP Jr, Perez AR. Postgastrectomy syndromes. In: Moody FG, Carey LC, Jones RS, et al, editors. Surgical treatment of digestive disease. Chicago: Year Book Medical Publishers; 1986. p. 264–73.
2. Wells CA, MacPhee IW. The afferent-loop syndrome: bilious regurgitation after subtotal gastrectomy and its relief. Lancet 1952;2(6747):1189–93.
3. Ritchie WP Jr. Alkaline reflux gastritis. An objective assessment of its diagnosis and treatment. Ann Surg 1980;192(3):288–98.
4. Gustavsson S, Kelly KA, Melton LJ 3rd, et al. Trends in peptic ulcer surgery. A population-based study in Rochester, Minnesota, 1956-1985. Gastroenterology 1988;94(3):688–94.
5. Bardhan KD, Royston C. Time, change and peptic ulcer disease in Rotherham, UK. Dig Liver Dis 2008;40(7):540–6.
6. Smith BR, Stabile BE. Emerging trends in peptic ulcer disease and damage control surgery in the *H. pylori* era. Am Surg 2005;71(9):797–801.
7. Wainess RM, Dimick JB, Upchurch GR Jr, et al. Epidemiology of surgically treated gastric cancer in the United States, 1988-2000. J Gastrointest Surg 2003;7(7):879–83.
8. Jemal A, Siegel R, Xu J, et al. Cancer statistics, 2010. CA Cancer J Clin 2010; 60(5):277–300.
9. Loffeld RJ. Prevalence of upper abdominal complaints in patients who have undergone partial gastrectomy. Can J Gastroenterol 2000;14(8):681–4.
10. Mine S, Sano T, Tsutsumi K, et al. Large-scale investigation into dumping syndrome after gastrectomy for gastric cancer. J Am Coll Surg 2010;211(5): 628–36.
11. Pedrazzani C, Marrelli D, Rampone B, et al. Postoperative complications and functional results after subtotal gastrectomy with Billroth II reconstruction for primary gastric cancer. Dig Dis Sci 2007;52(8):1757–63.
12. Livingston EH. The incidence of bariatric surgery has plateaued in the U.S. Am J Surg 2010;200(3):378–85.
13. Liedman B, Andersson H, Bosaeus I, et al. Changes in body composition after gastrectomy: results of a controlled, prospective clinical trial. World J Surg 1997;21(4):416–20 [discussion: 420–21].
14. Zittel TT, Zeeb B, Maier GW, et al. High prevalence of bone disorders after gastrectomy. Am J Surg 1997;174(4):431–8.

15. Melton LJ 3rd, Crowson CS, Khosla S, et al. Fracture risk after surgery for peptic ulcer disease: a population-based cohort study. Bone 1999;25(1):61–7.
16. Sipponen P, Härkönen M. Hypochlorhydric stomach: a risk condition for calcium malabsorption and osteoporosis? Scand J Gastroenterol 2010;45(2):133–8.
17. Nihei Z, Kojima K, Ichikawa W, et al. Chronological changes in bone mineral content following gastrectomy. Surg Today 1996;26(2):95–100.
18. Wetscher G, Redmond E, Watfah C, et al. Bone disorders following total gastrectomy. Dig Dis Sci 1994;39(12):2511–5.
19. Shiga K, Nishimukai M, Tomita F, et al. Ingestion of difructose anhydride III, a non-digestible disaccharide, improves postgastrectomy osteopenia in rats. Scand J Gastroenterol 2006;41(10):1165–73.
20. Shiga K, Hara H, Takahashi T, et al. Ingestion of water-soluble soybean fiber improves gastrectomy-induced calcium malabsorption and osteopenia in rats. Nutrition 2002;18(7–8):636–42.
21. Tan JC, Burns DL, Jones HR. Severe ataxia, myelopathy, and peripheral neuropathy due to acquired copper deficiency in a patient with history of gastrectomy. JPEN J Parenter Enteral Nutr 2006;30(5):446–50.
22. Everett CM, Matharu M, Gawler J. Neuropathy progressing to myeloneuropathy 20 years after partial gastrectomy. Neurology 2006;66(9):1451.
23. Beyan C, Beyan E, Kaptan K, et al. Post-gastrectomy anemia: evaluation of 72 cases with post-gastrectomy anemia. Hematology 2007;12(1):81–4.
24. Shiga K, Nishimukai M, Tomita F, et al. Ingestion of difructose anhydride III, a non-digestible disaccharide, prevents gastrectomy-induced iron malabsorption and anemia in rats. Nutrition 2006;22(7–8):786–93.
25. Hunt GC, Faigel DO. Endoscopic evaluation of patients with partial gastrectomy and iron deficiency. Dig Dis Sci 2002;47(3):641–4.
26. Le Blanc-Louvry I, Savoye G, Maillot C, et al. An impaired accommodation of the proximal stomach to a meal is associated with symptoms after distal gastrectomy. Am J Gastroenterol 2003;98(12):2642–7.
27. Ukleja A. Dumping syndrome: pathophysiology and treatment. Nutr Clin Pract 2005;20(5):517–25.
28. Yamamoto H, Mori T, Tsuchihashi H, et al. A possible role of GLP-1 in the pathophysiology of early dumping syndrome. Dig Dis Sci 2005;50(12):2263–7.
29. van der Kleij FG, Vecht J, Lamers CB, et al. Diagnostic value of dumping provocation in patients after gastric surgery. Scand J Gastroenterol 1996;31(12):1162–6.
30. Nunobe S, Okaro A, Sasako M, et al. Billroth 1 versus Roux-en-Y reconstructions: a quality-of-life survey at 5 years. Int J Clin Oncol 2007;12(6):433–9.
31. Li-Ling J, Irving M. Therapeutic value of octreotide for patients with severe dumping syndrome–a review of randomised controlled trials. Postgrad Med J 2001;77(909):441–2.
32. Arts J, Caenepeel P, Bisschops R, et al. Efficacy of the long-acting repeatable formulation of the somatostatin analogue octreotide in postoperative dumping. Clin Gastroenterol Hepatol 2009;7(4):432–7.
33. Penning C, Vecht J, Masclee AA. Efficacy of depot long-acting release octreotide therapy in severe dumping syndrome. Aliment Pharmacol Ther 2005;22(10):963–9.
34. Didden P, Penning C, Masclee AA. Octreotide therapy in dumping syndrome: analysis of long-term results. Aliment Pharmacol Ther 2006;24(9):1367–75.
35. Vecht J, Lamers CB, Masclee AA. Long-term results of octreotide-therapy in severe dumping syndrome. Clin Endocrinol (Oxf) 1999;51(5):619–24.

36. Imhof A, Schneemann M, Schaffner A, et al. Reactive hypoglycaemia due to late dumping syndrome: successful treatment with acarbose. Swiss Med Wkly 2001; 131(5–6):81–3.
37. Yamada M, Ohrui T, Asada M, et al. Acarbose attenuates hypoglycemia from dumping syndrome in an elderly man with gastrectomy. J Am Geriatr Soc 2005;53(2):358–9.
38. Nunobe S, Sasako M, Saka M, et al. Symptom evaluation of long-term postoperative outcomes after pylorus-preserving gastrectomy for early gastric cancer. Gastric Cancer 2007;10(3):167–72.
39. Ishikawa K, Arita T, Ninomiya S, et al. Outcome of segmental gastrectomy versus distal gastrectomy for early gastric cancer. World J Surg 2007;31(11): 2204–7.
40. Katsube T, Konnno S, Murayama M, et al. Gastric emptying after pylorus-preserving gastrectomy: assessment using the 13C-acetic acid breath test. Hepatogastroenterology 2007;54(74):639–42.
41. Nakane Y, Michiura T, Sakuramoto K, et al. Evaluation of the preserved function of the remnant stomach in pylorus preserving-gastrectomy by gastric emptying scintigraphy. Gan To Kagaku Ryoho 2007;34(1):25–8 [in Japanese].
42. Richards WO, Golzarian J, Wasudev N, et al. Reverse phasic contractions are present in antiperistaltic jejunal limbs up to twenty-one years postoperatively. J Am Coll Surg 1994;178(6):557–63.
43. Sawyers JL, Herrington JL. Superiority of antiperistaltic jejunal segments in management of severe dumping syndrome. Ann Surg 1973;178(3):311–9.
44. Nakane Y, Michiura T, Inoue K, et al. Role of pyloroplasty after proximal gastrectomy for cancer. Hepatogastroenterology 2004;51(60):1867–71.
45. Tomita R, Tanjoh K, Fujisaki S. Novel operative technique for vagal nerve- and pyloric sphincter-preserving distal gastrectomy reconstructed by interposition of a 5 cm jejunal J pouch with a 3 cm jejunal conduit for early gastric cancer and postoperative quality of life 5 years after operation. World J Surg 2004; 28(8):766–74.
46. Braun H. Ueber die Gastro-enterostomie and Gleichzeutig Ausgefuhrte. Arch Klin Chir 1893;84:361.
47. Jung HJ, Lee JH, Ryu KW, et al. The influence of reconstruction methods on food retention phenomenon in the remnant stomach after a subtotal gastrectomy. J Surg Oncol 2008;98(1):11–4.
48. Kubo M, Sasako M, Gotoda T, et al. Endoscopic evaluation of the remnant stomach after gastrectomy: proposal for a new classification. Gastric Cancer 2002;5(2):83–9.
49. Speicher JE, Thirlby RC, Burggraaf J, et al. Results of completion gastrectomies in 44 patients with postsurgical gastric atony. J Gastrointest Surg 2009;13(5): 874–80.
50. Kojima K, Yamada H, Inokuchi M, et al. A comparison of Roux-en-Y and Billroth-I reconstruction after laparoscopy-assisted distal gastrectomy. Ann Surg 2008; 247(6):962–7.
51. Tu BL, Kelly KA. Surgical treatment of Roux stasis syndrome. J Gastrointest Surg 1999;3(6):613–7.
52. Cullen JJ, Eagon JC, Hould FS, et al. Ectopic jejunal pacemakers after jejunal transection and their relationship to transit. Am J Physiol 1995;268(6 Pt 1): G959–67.
53. Miedema BW, Kelly KA, Camilleri M, et al. Human gastric and jejunal transit and motility after Roux gastrojejunostomy. Gastroenterology 1992;103(4):1133–43.

54. Fukuhara K, Osugi H, Takada N, et al. Reconstructive procedure after distal gastrectomy for gastric cancer that best prevents duodenogastroesophageal reflux. World J Surg 2002;26(12):1452–7.
55. Krönert T, Kähler G, Adam G, et al. Fiber optic measurements with the Bilitec probe for quantifying bile reflux after aboral stomach resection. Zentralbl Chir 1998;123(3):239–44 [in German].
56. Osugi H, Fukuhara K, Takada N, et al. Reconstructive procedure after distal gastrectomy to prevent remnant gastritis. Hepatogastroenterology 2004;51(58): 1215–8.
57. Csendes A, Burgos AM, Smok G, et al. Latest results (12-21 years) of a prospective randomized study comparing Billroth II and Roux-en-Y anastomosis after a partial gastrectomy plus vagotomy in patients with duodenal ulcers. Ann Surg 2009;249(2):189–94.
58. Fukuhara K, Osugi H, Takada N, et al. Quantitative determinations of duodenogastric reflux, prevalence of *Helicobacter pylori* infection, and concentrations of interleukin-8. World J Surg 2003;27(5):567–70.
59. Namikawa T, Kitagawa H, Okabayashi T, et al. Roux-en-Y reconstruction is superior to Billroth I reconstruction in reducing reflux esophagitis after distal gastrectomy: special relationship with the angle of His. World J Surg 2010;34(5):1022–7.
60. Wu CC, Chen CY, Wu TC, et al. Cholelithiasis and cholecystitis after gastrectomy for gastric carcinoma: a comparison of lymphadenectomy of varying extent. Hepatogastroenterology 1995;42(6):867–72.
61. Turnage RH, Sarosi G, Cryer B, et al. Evaluation and management of patients with recurrent peptic ulcer disease after acid-reducing operations: a systematic review. J Gastrointest Surg 2003;7(5):606–26.
62. Lee YT, Sung JJ, Choi CL, et al. Ulcer recurrence after gastric surgery: is *Helicobacter pylori* the culprit? Am J Gastroenterol 1998;93(6):928–31.
63. Ingvar C, Adami HO, Enander LK, et al. Clinical results of reoperation after failed highly selective vagotomy. Am J Surg 1986;152(3):308–12.
64. Balfour DC. Factors influencing the life expectancy of patients operated on for gastric ulcer. Ann Surg 1922;76(3):405–8.
65. Helsingen N, Hillestad L. Cancer development in the gastric stump after partial gastrectomy for ulcer. Ann Surg 1956;143(2):173–9.
66. Krause U. Late prognosis after partial gastrectomy for ulcer; a follow-up study of 361 patients operated upon from 1905 to 1933. Acta Chir Scand 1958;114(5): 341–54.
67. Fischer AB, Graem N, Jensen OM. Risk of gastric cancer after Billroth II resection for duodenal ulcer. Br J Surg 1983;70(9):552–4.
68. Viste A, Bjørnestad E, Opheim P, et al. Risk of carcinoma following gastric operations for benign disease. A historical cohort study of 3470 patients. Lancet 1986; 2(8505):502–5.
69. Arnthorsson G, Tulinius H, Egilsson V, et al. Gastric cancer after gastrectomy. Int J Cancer 1988;42(3):365–7.
70. Lundegårdh G, Adami HO, Helmick C, et al. Stomach cancer after partial gastrectomy for benign ulcer disease. N Engl J Med 1988;319(4):195–200.
71. Fisher SG, Davis F, Nelson R, et al. A cohort study of stomach cancer risk in men after gastric surgery for benign disease. J Natl Cancer Inst 1993;85(16):1303–10.
72. Miwa K, Hasegawa H, Fujimura T, et al. Duodenal reflux through the pylorus induces gastric adenocarcinoma in the rat. Carcinogenesis 1992;13(12):2313–6.
73. Ruddell WS, Bone ES, Hill MJ, et al. Gastric-juice nitrite. A risk factor for cancer in the hypochlorhydric stomach? Lancet 1976;2(7994):1037–9.

74. Greenlee HB, Vivit R, Paez J, et al. Bacterial flora of the jejunum following peptic ulcer surgery. Arch Surg 1971;102(4):260–5.
75. Schlag P, Böckler R, Ulrich H, et al. Are nitrite and N-nitroso compounds in gastric juice risk factors for carcinoma in the operated stomach? Lancet 1980;1(8171): 727–9.
76. Tanigawa N, Nomura E, Lee SW, et al, Society for the Study of Postoperative Morbidity after Gastrectomy. Current state of gastric stump carcinoma in Japan: based on the results of a nationwide survey. World J Surg 2010;34(7):1540–7.
77. Caygill CP, Hill MJ, Hall CN, et al. Increased risk of cancer at multiple sites after gastric surgery for peptic ulcer. Gut 1987;28(8):924–8.
78. Ross AH, Smith MA, Anderson JR, et al. Late mortality after surgery for peptic ulcer. N Engl J Med 1982;307(9):519–22.
79. Schweizer W, Blunschi T, Seiler C. Postgastrectomy symptoms after partial stomach resection: Billroth I vs. Billroth II vs. reconstruction with roux-Y-loop. Helv Chir Acta 1994 Apr;60(4):665–9 [in German].
80. Ishikawa M, Kitayama J, Kaizaki S, et al. Prospective randomized trial comparing Billroth I and Roux-en-Y procedures after distal gastrectomy for gastric carcinoma. World J Surg 2005;29(11):1415–20 [discussion: 1421].
81. Hunt CJ. Construction of food pouch from segment of jejunum as substitute for stomach in total gastrectomy. AMA Arch Surg 1952;64(5):601–8.
82. Svedlund J, Sullivan M, Liedman B, et al. Quality of life after gastrectomy for gastric carcinoma: controlled study of reconstructive procedures. World J Surg 1997;21(4):422–33.
83. Schmitz R, Moser KH, Treckmann J. Quality of life after prograde jejunum interposition with and without pouch. A prospective study of stomach cancer patients on the reservoir as a reconstruction principle after total gastrectomy. Chirurg 1994; 65(4):326–32 [in German].
84. Iivonen MK, Mattila JJ, Nordback IH, et al. Long-term follow-up of patients with jejunal pouch reconstruction after total gastrectomy. A randomized prospective study. Scand J Gastroenterol 2000;35(7):679–85.
85. Zhang JZ, Lu HS, Wu XY, et al. Influence of different procedures of alimentary tract reconstruction after total gastrectomy for gastric cancer on the nutrition and metabolism of patients: a prospective clinical study. Zhonghua Yi Xue Za Zhi 2003;83(17):1475–8 [in Chinese].
86. Kono K, Iizuka H, Sekikawa T, et al. Improved quality of life with jejunal pouch reconstruction after total gastrectomy. Am J Surg 2003;185(2):150–4.
87. Fein M, Fuchs KH, Thalheimer A, et al. Long-term benefits of Roux-en-Y pouch reconstruction after total gastrectomy: a randomized trial. Ann Surg 2008; 247(5):759–65.
88. Nakane Y, Okumura S, Akehira K, et al. Jejunal pouch reconstruction after total gastrectomy for cancer. A randomized controlled trial. Ann Surg 1995 Jul; 222(1):27–35.
89. Bozzetti F, Bonfanti G, Castellani R, et al. Comparing reconstruction with Roux-en-Y to a pouch following total gastrectomy. J Am Coll Surg 1996;183(3):243–8.
90. Schwarz A, Büchler M, Usinger K, et al. Importance of the duodenal passage and pouch volume after total gastrectomy and reconstruction with the Ulm pouch: prospective randomized clinical study. World J Surg 1996;20(1):60–6 [discussion: 66–67].
91. Svedlund J, Sullivan M, Liedman B, et al. Long term consequences of gastrectomy for patient's quality of life: the impact of reconstructive techniques. Am J Gastroenterol 1999;94(2):438–45.

92. Gertler R, Rosenberg R, Feith M, et al. Pouch vs. no pouch following total gastrectomy: meta-analysis and systematic review. Am J Gastroenterol 2009;104(11):2838–51.
93. Eypasch E, Williams JI, Wood-Dauphinee S, et al. Gastrointestinal Quality of Life Index: development, validation and application of a new instrument. Br J Surg 1995;82(2):216–22.
94. Fuchs KH, Thiede A, Engemann R, et al. Reconstruction of the food passage after total gastrectomy: randomized trial. World J Surg 1995;19(5):698–705 [discussion: 705–6].
95. Nakane Y, Michiura T, Inoue K, et al. A randomized clinical trial of pouch reconstruction after total gastrectomy for cancer: which is the better technique, Roux-en-Y or interposition? Hepatogastroenterology 2001;48(39):903–7.

Miscellaneous Disorders and Their Management in Gastric Surgery: Volvulus, Carcinoid, Lymphoma, Gastric Varices, and Gastric Outlet Obstruction

Stephen A. Dada, MD, George M. Fuhrman, MD*

KEYWORDS

• Volvulus • Carcinoid • Lymphoma • Gastric varices
• Gastric outlet obstruction

The final article in this issue focuses on less common diseases that surgeons are called on for management options. These five topics—volvulus, carcinoid, lymphoma, gastric varices, and gastric outlet obstruction (GOO) from peptic ulcer disease—are frequently used to evaluate surgical knowledge. Knowledge of these topics is useful for residents preparing for an in-training examination or board certification. Patients with these diseases require multidisciplinary management with oncologists and/or gastroenterologists, and mastery of these topics allows surgeons to effectively participate in the multidisciplinary care of these patients and advocate for surgical management when appropriate.

GASTRIC VOLVULUS

Gastric volvulus is a rare condition defined as an abnormal rotation of all or part of the stomach. Volvulus may occur along the vertical axis, mesoaxial torsion, or more commonly along an organoaxial direction. The less common mesoaxial torsion is associated with a less than 180° twist and the stomach situated below the diaphragm;

Department of Surgery, Atlanta Medical Center, Box 423, 303 Parkway, NE, Atlanta, GA 30312, USA

* Corresponding author.

E-mail address: George.fuhrman@tenethealth.com

Surg Clin N Am 91 (2011) 1123–1130
doi:10.1016/j.suc.2011.06.011 surgical.theclinics.com
0039-6109/11/$ – see front matter © 2011 Elsevier Inc. All rights reserved.

it is not discussed further. Organoaxial torsion patients have a diaphragmatic defect and a greater than 180° torsion and demand immediate surgical attention. The diagnosis of volvulus should be suspected based on the findings of Borchardt triad, initially reported more than a century ago, that include severe upper abdominal pain, retching with little vomitus, and inability to pass a nasogtastric tube for decompression.[1] Not all patients with gastric volvulus demonstrate acute obstructive symptoms requiring emergency surgery; instead, a chronic condition that is minimally or asymptomatic might be discovered incidentally on a radiographic study performed for an unrelated purpose. Often the first tests performed in patients with chest or abdominal complaints are plain films that may demonstrate an intrathoracic stomach. Upper gastrointestinal (GI) contrast study has remained the gold standard and if performed with the stomach in the twisted state depicts an upside-down stomach.[2] CT scanning showing a double bubble with a transition line is gaining popularity as the imaging modality of choice.[3] In the acute setting with severe symptoms, upper GI and CT scanning sensitivity can be limited by a patient's inability to tolerate oral contrast material. Even on a CT without oral contrast, the clearly intrathoracic twisted stomach is evident.

The treatment of gastric volvulus is surgical and the goal of surgical therapy is reduction, decompression, débridement, and prevention of recurrence. Through a midline laparotomy, the stomach is reduced and assessed for viability. The stomach's rich vascularity makes nonviability uncommon. Nonviable portions of the stomach are resected and a tube gastrostomy tube or suture gastropexy can be performed to prevent recurrence. Gastrostomy tubes placed in these situations are ideally situated in the left midabdomen, lower than where a typical open gastrostomy is placed to help fix the typically dilated stomach within the abdominal cavity. Care should be taken to place the tube low on the abdominal wall; however, undue tension created by pexing the stomach too low on the abdomen can result in dislodgement of the tube with intraperitoneal leak.[4,5] Surgery for acute gastric volvulus is a surgical emergency and mortality is closely associated to delay in diagnosis. Surgery for chronic volvulus is elective and is performed to alleviate symptoms and prevent future complications. Minimally invasive techniques have been described and may reduce the morbidity associated with the open procedure.[6,7] Because associated diaphragmatic defects should be expected, surgeons who use a laparoscopic approach must be facile with advanced techniques, including mesh placement and suture fixation. Endoscopic reduction has been described in selected groups of patients.[8–10] Because of the increased risk of gastric perforation during endoscopic reduction, this technique should be limited to patients medically unfit for surgery. The outcome for gastric volvulus is dependent on timely diagnosis and proper management. The reported mortality rate from acute gastric volvulus is 15% to 20% and for chronic gastric volvulus is 0% to 13%.[4,11]

GASTRIC CARCINOID

Gastric carcinoid tumors are rare and comprise approximately 8.7% to 30% of GI carcinoids and approximately 1% of all gastric neoplasms.[12] Also known as neuroendocrine tumors, they are derived from the enterochromaffin cells of the gastric corpus that mediate the secretion of histamine, which stimulates their unique receptors on parietal cells to stimulate acid production. The tumors are submucosal and most commonly occur in the fundus or antrum of the stomach. Three subtypes are described. Type I lesions are the most common (approximately 80% of the total) and are associated with the hypergastrinemia found in chronic atrophic gastritis, pernicious anemia, autoimmune atrophic gastritis, and chronic antiacid treatment with histamine blockers and proton pump inhibitors. Hypergastrinemia results in enterochromaffin cell hyperplasia, which may give rise to type I gastric carcinoids.[13] Tumors are more commonly seen in women over age 50 and usually small in size and asymptomatic at time of diagnosis. Type II lesions (approximately 5% of the total) are associated with gastrinomas, are equally distributed in men and women, and can be found in patients with Zollinger-Ellison syndrome or in patients with multiple endocrine neoplasia, type I.[14,15] Type III (approximately 15% of the total) gastric carcinoids occur sporadically, presenting as solitary large tumors, and are not associated with hypergastrinemia. They occur more commonly in men and have high malignant potential; approximately 50% of patients have metastatic disease at the time of diagnosis. Biochemical analysis includes measuring 24-hour urine levels of 5-hydroxyindoleacetic acid, which is a serotonin metabolite. A pentagastrin provocative test may be performed if the 24-hour urine levels of 5-hydroxyindoleacetic acid is inconclusive. Because of their small size and asymptomatic nature, most carcinoid tumors are found incidentally during esophagogastroduodenoscopy performed for other reasons. Endoscopic ultrasonography can be used to determine size and depth of the lesion. CT and MRI can be used to identify the primary tumor, local lymph node involvement, and metastatic spread. Somatostatin receptor scintigraphy (95% sensitive) is used to localize carcinoid tumors not seen on other imaging modalities. Type I lesions less than 1 cm and confined to the mucosa may be removed endoscopically. Surveillance endoscopy is recommended to monitor for recurrence. Antrectomy is recommended for type I gastric carcinoids when there are more than 5 lesions or 1 lesion greater than 1 cm.[16] For older patients discovered to have an indolent disease, however, such as a type I gastric carcinoid, a valid argument can be made for consideration of observation and stopping antiacid hypergastrinemia causing medications if a patient's symptoms allow. Type II tumors less than 1 cm may be treated endoscopically[16]; however, multiple lesions and tumors greater than 1 cm should be removed by partial gastrectomy. Because type III lesions often present with local lymph node involvement, treatment includes partial or total gastrectomy with extended lymph node resection.[17] Type I gastric carcinoids are generally benign and slow growing and have an excellent 5-year survival rate of greater than 95%. Type II lesions are of intermediate malignant potential and overall have a good prognosis, 70% to 90% five year disease free survival. Type III lesions have the most malignant potential and a 5-year survival rate of less than 35%.[18] The differentiation of type I from type III carcinoids is critically important because an aggressive approach to type III lesions is indicated whereas nonoperative observational management may be appropriate for type I lesions. A larger lesion that cannot be explained by a condition or medication associated with gastrin excess should be approached like a gastric adenocarcinoma, with radiographic staging and consideration of aggressive local and regional resections.

GASTRIC LYMPHOMA

The stomach is the most common site of primary extranodal non-Hodgkin lymphoma (NHL) of the GI tract. The two main histologic subtypes are mucosa-associated lymphoid tissue (MALT) NHL and diffuse large B-cell NHL. Chronic gastritis associated with *Helicobacter pylori* infection has been shown to be the cause of MALT and atrophic gastritis has been proposed as a risk factor for diffuse large B-cell NHL. As with most patients with NHL, there is a male predominance. Symptoms are nonspecific and include abdominal pain, dyspepsia, nausea, vomiting, and anorexia. Constitutional symptoms are uncommon. Upper GI bleeding may be the presentation in up to 20% to 30% of patients[19]; gastric obstruction and perforation occur less frequently. Diagnosis is obtained by endoscopic biopsy. Gastric MALT is characterized by the presence of lymphoepithelial lesions that are formed by invasion of single glands by aggregates of neoplastic cells with centrocyte morphology.[20] Lymphoma diffuse large B-cell is characterized by a centroblastic morphology.[21] Staging procedures for primary gastric lymphomas include laboratory analysis for lactate dehydrogenase; β2-macroglobulin; CT of the abdomen, pelvis, and chest; and bone marrow aspiration and biopsy. Positron emission tomography has been shown beneficial for diffuse large B-cell to examine the volume of disease at time of diagnosis.[22] Three staging systems are described and used to guide therapy: the Ann Arbor classification system, the Lugano staging system, and more recently the Paris staging system (**Table 1**). The Paris staging system is a modified TNM classification system that describes the depth of tumor infiltration the extent of nodal involvement and the extent of local tissue infiltration by lymphoma.[23]

Treatment of low-grade MALT lymphomas confined to the stomach can be accomplished by eradication of *H pylori* with antibiotics. Complete remission can be seen in up to 70% of patients.[24] Relapse is associated with *H pylori* reinfection and, therefore, endoscopic follow-up is recommended. For patients unresponsive to antibiotics or for the subset of *H pylori*–negative cases (approximately 10%), radiation therapy alone in patients with early stages (I and II) can achieve greater than 95% complete response rates.[25] If patients have contraindications to radiation therapy, a single-agent chemotherapy (rituximab) can also be used.

Table 1
Comparison of Lugano, Ann Arbor, and Paris staging systems in primary GI lymphomas

Lugano Staging System for Gastrointestinal Lymphomas		Ann Arbor Stage	TNM Staging System Adapted for Gastric Lymphoma	Tumor Extension
Stage I_E	Confined to G1 tract			
	I_{E1} = mucosa, submucosa	1_E	T1 N0 M0	Mucosa, submucosa
	I_{E2} = muscularis propria, serosa	I_E	T2 N0 M0	Muscularis propria
		I_E	T3 N0 M0	Serosa
Stage II_E	Extending into abdomen			
	II_{E1}= local nodal Involvement	II_E	T1-3 N1 M0	Perigastric lymph nodes
	II_{E2}= distant nodal involvement	II_E	T1-S N2 M0	More distant regional lymph nodes
Stage II_E	Penetration of serosa to involve adjacent organs or tissues	II_E	T4 N0 M0	Invasion of adjacent structures
Stage III-IV	Disseminated extranodal involvement or concomitant supradiaphragmatic nodal involvement	III_E IV	T1-4 N3 M0 T1-4 N0-3 mL	Lymph nodes on both sides of the diaphragm/distant metastases (eg, bone marrow or additional extra nodal sites)

From Yahalom J. Extranodal marginal zone B-cell lymphoma of mucosa-asssociated lymphoid tissue (MALT lymphoma). In: Hoppe R, Mauch PM, Armitage JO, et al, editors. Non-Hodgkin's lymphomas. Philadelphia: Lippincott; 2004. p. 352; with permission.

Advanced-stage MALT lymphomas (stage III and IV) are rare and, because of its indolent nature, chemotherapy is not curative; therefore, asymptomatic patients can be observed without treatment. Indications for systemic therapy include candidate for clinical trial, symptomatic disease, GI bleeding, threatened end-organ function, bulky disease, steady progression, and patient preference.

Treatment of diffuse gastric large B-cell lymphoma is rituximab plus chemotherapy with anthracycline-based regimens (cyclophosphamide, vincristine [Oncovin], hydroxydaunorubicin, and prednisone [CHOP]; cyclophosphamide, epirubicin, vincristine [Oncovin], and prednisone [CEOP]; and cyclophosphamide, mitoxantrone [Novantrone], vincristine [Oncovin], and prednisone [CNOP]).

Surgery for primary gastric lymphoma is indicated for the following: primary radical treatment, severe bleeding or perforation, and as palliative treatment.[26] Because surgery is associated with higher rates of morbidity when compared with radiation alone and chemotherapy alone, the treatment strategy has shifted toward organ preservation. The first-line chemotherapy regimens are combination chemotherapy that includes rituximab and CHOP (R-CHOP) or bendamustine and rituximab. Despite its aggressive nature, the 5-year survival rate of diffuse gastric large B-cell lymphoma is good, ranging from 73% to 90% after primary systemic therapy.[26] The 5-year survival rate for patients with low-grade gastric MALT is greater than 91%, with 5-year survival rates ranging from 50% to 70% in patients with high-grade gastric MALT tumors.[27]

ISOLATED GASTRIC VARICES

Isolated gastric varices occur in patients with segmental or left-sided portal hypertension due to splenic vein thrombosis. This condition must be differentiated from gastric varices seen in association with esophageal varices in the setting of portal hypertension. The management of patients with combined gastric and esophageal varices should be focused on the treatment of the underlying portal hypertension and is not discussed further in this article. Isolated gastric varices result from benign and malignant pancreatic pathology that cause splenic vein thrombosis. Direct tumor extension or the fibrosis associated with chronic inflammatory conditions can obstruct the splenic vein, causing thrombosis. Continued arterial flow to the spleen engorges the gland, resulting in splenomegaly that can only decompress through the normally small-caliber short gastric veins. These small veins dilate and can ulcerate through the gastric mucosa and cause upper GI bleeding. Patients with gastric varices develop large dilated submucosal veins in the stomach and may present with hematemesis, hematochezia, or melena.

The risk of bleeding from isolated gastric varices is low when compared with that of gastroesophageal varices. When isolated gastric varices are incidentally detected at endoscopy and proved the result of splenic vein thrombosis, treatment is unnecessary due to a low risk of bleeding.[28,29] When upper GI endoscopy is used to evaluate a bleeding patient, however, the finding of gastric varices without esophageal varices is virtually diagnostic of splenic vein thrombosis. Abdominal imaging with contrast-enhanced CT or MRI is essential to evaluate the pancreas to differentiate benign from malignant etiologies.[30] Laboratory analysis should include complete blood count, coagulation factors, and liver function test, and cancer antigen 19-9 levels may be helpful if benign versus malignant causes are not apparent on imaging studies. Initial treatment should focus on airway protection followed by large bore venous access and resuscitation with blood products. The treatment of choice for bleeding isolated gastric varices is splenectomy, which effectively eliminates the collateral outflow.[31,32]

When bleeding gastric varices results in splenic vein thrombosis from pancreatic carcinoma of the body or tail of the gland, curative resection is highly unlikely and splenectomy in this situation should be judiciously used.[33]

BENIGN GASTRIC OUTLET OBSTRUCTION

Patients with GOO may have either benign or malignant causes of blockage. In general, patients with malignant causes of GOO have advanced disease, a limited life expectancy, and imaging studies that demonstrate widespread metastases.[34] When patients have signs and symptoms of GOO without evidence of metastatic cancer, endoscopy is typically performed to determine whether the cause of obstruction is benign or malignant. The distally obstructed stomach that does not permit easy passage of the endoscope may not allow for access to the tumor for biopsy. Therefore, surgeons should not be fooled by benign biopsies that may reflect the difficulty with sampling the tumor and should rely on abdominal imaging in addition to endoscopic findings to distinguish cancer from benign causes of obstruction. The topic of surgery in the setting of stage IV cancer is discussed by Patel and Kooby in the article on gastric adenocarcinoma elsewhere in this issue and not discussed further in this article. When imaging demonstrates isolated GOO and endoscopy fails to document cancer, patients should be evaluated for either surgical or endoscopic management of what is most likely a benign cause of obstruction, most frequently a result of chronic neglected peptic ulcer disease. Although balloon dilation and medical management of GOO, including *H pylori* eradication, have been reported, the ultimate need for surgery increases with longer follow-up because some patients who initially respond to nonoperative management relapse and ultimately require surgery.[35,36] Gibson and colleagues[37] reported a surgical series of 24 patients treated by surgery for GOO from ulcer disease. This group from Memphis found that only one-third of patients were *H pylori* positive, nonsteroidal anti-inflammatory drugs were a common cause of GOO from ulcer disease, and that all but one patient was dramatically improved by surgery. The choice of operation is either resection of the obstructed antrum and pylorus or bypass. Because a gastrojejunal bypass is ulcerogenic with acid-rich secretions bathing an unprotected jejunum, resection is preferred as long as the proximal duodenum can be safely divided and closed. Surgeons' confidence in their ability to achieve a satisfactory duodenal closure drives the intraoperative decision as to whether resection or bypass is most appropriate. Ulcerogenic bypass procedures are preferred to the morbidity associated with the complications of a difficult duodenal stump and the potential for a leak and development of a duodenocutaneous fistula. Patients treated by gastrojejunostomy as a bypass of a benign obstructed stomach require acid reduction in the form of vagotomy or lifelong medication. Because the development of GOO by ulcer occurs over a protracted time course with symptoms that likely are ignored by patients, many of these patients are noncompliant and may do better with vagotomy instead of relying on lifelong medication.

REFERENCES

1. Borchardt M. Aus Patholoe und therapie des magenvolvulus. Arch Klin Chir 1904;74:243 [in German].
2. Levine ML, Gelberg B. Gastric mucosal disruption (fissuring) as a sign of impending perforation in a patient with gastric volvulus. Gastrointest Endosc 1993;39:214–5.

3. Gourgiotis S, Vougas V, Germanos S, et al. Acute gastric volvulus: diagnosis and management over 10 years. Dig Surg 2006;23(3):169–72.
4. Haas O, Rat P, Christophe M, et al. Surgical results of intrathoracic gastric volvulus complicating hiatal hernia. Br J Surg 1990;77:1379.
5. Carlson MA, Condon RE, Ludwig KA, et al. Management of intrathoracic stomach with polypropylene mesh prosthesis reinforced transabdominal hiatus hernia repair. J Am Coll Surg 1998;187(3):227–30.
6. Palanivelu C, Rangarajan M, Shetty AR, et al. Laparoscopic suture gastropexy for gastric volvulus: a report of 14 cases. Surg Endosc 2007;21(6):863–6.
7. Katkhouda N, Mavor E, Achanta K, et al. Laparoscopic repair of chronic intrathoracic gastric volvulus. Surgery 2000;5:784–90.
8. Hani MB. A combined laparoscopic and endoscopic approach to acute gastric volvulus associated with traumatic diaphragmatic hernia. Surg Laparosc Endosc Percutan Tech 2008;18(2):151–4.
9. Kulkarni K, Nagler J. Emergency endoscopic reduction of a gastric volvulus. Endoscopy 2007;39:E173.
10. Baudet JS, Armengol-Miro JR, Medina C. Percutaneous endoscopic gastrostomy as a treatment for chronic gastric volvulus. Endoscopy 1997;29(2):147–8.
11. Hsu YC, Perng CL, Chen CK, et al. Conservative management of chronic gastric volvulus: 44 cases over 5 years. World J Surg 2010;16(33):4200–5.
12. Modlin IM, Lye KD, Kidd MA. 5-Decade analysis of 13,715 carcinoid tumors. Cancer 2003;97:934–59.
13. Landry CS, McMasters KM, Scroggins CR, et al. A proposed staging system for gastric carcinoid tumors based on analysis of 1,543 patients. Ann Surg Oncol 2009;16(1):51–60.
14. Peghini PL, Annibale B, Azzoni C, et al. Effect of chronic hypergastrinemia on human enterochromaffin cells: insights from patients with sporadic gastrinoma. Gastroenterology 2002;123(1):68–85.
15. Berna MJ, Annibale B, Marignani M, et al. A prospective study of gastric carcinoids and enterochromaffin-like cell changes in multiple endocrine Neoplasia type 1 and Zollinger-Ellison syndrome: identification of risk factors. J Clin Endocrinol Metab 2008;93(5):1582–91.
16. Borch K, Ahrén B, Ahlam H. Gastric carcinoids: biologic behavior and prognosis after differentiated treatment in relation to type. Ann Surg 2005;242:64–73.
17. Modlin IM, Lye KD, Kidd M. Carcinoid tumors of the stomach. Surg Oncol 2003; 12:153–72.
18. Modlin IM, Kidd M, Latich I. Current status of gastrointestinal carcinoids. Gastroenterology 2005;128:1717–51.
19. Koch P, del Valle F, Berdel WE, et al. Primary gastrointestinal non-Hodgkins lymphoma: anatomic and histologic distribution, clinical features, and survival data of 371 patients registered in the German Multicenter study GIT NHL 01/92. J Clin Oncol 2001;19:3861–73.
20. Papadaki L, Wotherspoon AC, Isaacson PG. The lymphoepithelial lesion of gastric low-grade B -cell lymphoma of mucosa-associated lymphoid tissue (MALT): an ultrastructural study. Histopathology 1992;21:415–21.
21. Isaacson PG, Du MQ. Gastrointestinal lymphoma: where morphology meets molecular biology. J Pathol 2005;205:255–74.
22. Elstrom R, Guan L, Baker G, et al. Utility of FDG-PET scanning in lymphoma by WHO classification. Blood 2003;101:3875–6.
23. Rouskone FA, Dragosics B, Morgner A, et al. Paris staging system for primary gastrointestinal lymphomas. Gut 2003;52:912–3.

24. Bayerdorffer E, Neubauser A, Rudolph B, et al. Regression of primary gastric lymphoma tissue type after cure of Helicobacter pylori infection. MALT Lymphoma Study Group. Lancet 1995;345:1591–4.
25. Schechter NR, Portlock CS, Yahalom J. Treatment of mucosa-associated lymphoid tissue lymphoma of the stomach with radiation alone. J Clin Oncol 1998;16: 1916–21.
26. Ferreri AJ, Cordio S, Ponzoni M, et al. Non-surgical treatment with primary chemotherapy, with or without radiation therapy, of stage I-II high grade gastric lymphoma. Leuk Lymphoma 1999;33:531–41.
27. Al-Akwaa AM, Siddiqui N, Al-Mofleh IA. Primay gastric lymphoma. World J Gastroenterol 2004;10:5–11.
28. Weber SM, Rikkers LF. Splenic vein thrombosis and gastrointestinal bleeding in chronic pancreatitis. World J Surg 2003;27(11):1271–4.
29. Heider TR, Azeem S, Galanko JA, et al. The natural history of pancreatitis-induced splenic vein thrombosis. Ann Surg 2004;239(6):876–80.
30. Ryan BM, Stockbrugger RW, Ryan JM. A pathophysiologic gastroenterologic and radiologic approach to the management of gastric varices. Gastroenterology 2004;126:1175–89.
31. Sutton JP, Yarborough DY, Richards JT. Isolated splenic vein occlusion. Arch Surg 1970;100:623–30.
32. Sakorafas GH, Sarr MG, Farley DR, et al. The significance of sinistral portal hyper-tertension complicating chronic pancreatitis. Am J Surg 2000;179:129–33.
33. Smith TA, Brand EJ. Pancreatic cancer presenting as bleeding gastric varices. J Clin Gastroenterol 2001;32(5):444–7.
34. Schmidt C, Gerdes H, Hawkins W, et al. A prospective observational study examining quality of life in patients with malignant gastric outlet obstruction. Am J Surg 2009;198(1):92–9.
35. Lam YH, Lau JY, Fung TM, et al. Endoscopic balloon dilation for benign gastric outlet obstruction with and without Helicobacter pylori infection. Gastrointest Endosc 2004;60(2):229–33.
36. Cherian PT, Cherian S, Singh P. Long-term follow-up of patients with gastric outlet obstruction related to peptic ulcer disease treated with endoscopic balloon dilatation and drug therapy. Gastrointest Endosc 2007;66(3):491–7.
37. Gibson JB, Behrman SW, Fabian TC, et al. Gastric outlet obstruction resulting from peptic ulcer disease requiring surgical intervention is infrequently associated with Helicobacter pylori infection. J Am Coll Surg 2000;191(1):32–7.

Index

Note: Page numbers of article titles are in **boldface** type.

Surg Clin N Am 91 (2011) 1131–1138
doi:10.1016/S0039-6109(11)00112-5

0039-6109/11/$ – see front matter © 2011 Elsevier Inc. All rights reserved.

H

I

L

M

N

P

R

United States Postal Service

Statement of Ownership, Management, and Circulation
(All Periodicals Publications Except Requestor Publications)

1. Publication Title: Surgical Clinics of North America
2. Publication Number: 5 2 9 - 8 0 0
3. Filing Date: 9/16/11
4. Issue Frequency: Feb, Apr, Jun, Aug, Oct, Dec
5. Number of Issues Published Annually: 6
6. Annual Subscription Price: $311.00
7. Complete Mailing Address of Known Office of Publication (*Not printer*) (*Street, city, county, state, and ZIP+4®*)
   Elsevier Inc.
   360 Park Avenue South
   New York, NY 10010-1710

   Contact Person: Stephen Bushing
   Telephone (Include area code): 215-239-3688
8. Complete Mailing Address of Headquarters or General Business Office of Publisher (*Not printer*)
   Elsevier Inc., 360 Park Avenue South, New York, NY 10010-1710
9. Full Names and Complete Mailing Addresses of Publisher, Editor, and Managing Editor (*Do not leave blank*)
   Publisher (*Name and complete mailing address*)
   Kim Murphy, Elsevier, Inc., 1600 John F. Kennedy Blvd. Suite 1800, Philadelphia, PA 19103-2899
   Editor (*Name and complete mailing address*)
   John Vassallo, Elsevier, Inc., 1600 John F. Kennedy Blvd. Suite 1800, Philadelphia, PA 19103-2899
   Managing Editor (*Name and complete mailing address*)
   Barbara Cohen-Kligerman, Elsevier, Inc., 1600 John F. Kennedy Blvd. Suite 1800, Philadelphia, PA 19103-2899
10. Owner (*Do not leave blank. If the publication is owned by a corporation, give the name and address of the corporation immediately followed by the names and addresses of all stockholders owning or holding 1 percent or more of the total amount of stock. If not owned by a corporation, give the names and addresses of the individual owners. If owned by a partnership or other unincorporated firm, give its name and address as well as those of each individual owner. If the publication is published by a nonprofit organization, give its name and address.*)

Full Name	Complete Mailing Address
Wholly owned subsidiary of	4520 East-West Highway
Reed/Elsevier, US holdings	Bethesda, MD 20814

11. Known Bondholders, Mortgagees, and Other Security Holders Owning or Holding 1 Percent or More of Total Amount of Bonds, Mortgages, or Other Securities. If none, check box → ☐ None

Full Name	Complete Mailing Address
N/A	

12. Tax Status (*For completion by nonprofit organizations authorized to mail at nonprofit rates*) (*Check one*)
    The purpose, function, and nonprofit status of this organization and the exempt status for federal income tax purposes:
    ☐ Has Not Changed During Preceding 12 Months
    ☐ Has Changed During Preceding 12 Months (*Publisher must submit explanation of change with this statement*)

PS Form 3526, September 2007 (Page 1 of 3 (Instructions Page 3)) PSN 7530-01-000-9931 **PRIVACY NOTICE**: See our Privacy policy in www.usps.com

13. Publication Title: Surgical Clinics of North America
14. Issue Date for Circulation Data Below: August 2011

15. Extent and Nature of Circulation			Average No. Copies Each Issue During Preceding 12 Months	No. Copies of Single Issue Published Nearest to Filing Date
a. Total Number of Copies (*Net press run*)			3337	2768
b. Paid Circulation (By Mail and Outside the Mail)	(1)	Mailed Outside-County Paid Subscriptions Stated on PS Form 3541. (*Include paid distribution above nominal rate, advertiser's proof copies, and exchange copies*)	1278	1146
	(2)	Mailed In-County Paid Subscriptions Stated on PS Form 3541 (*Include paid distribution above nominal rate, advertiser's proof copies, and exchange copies*)		
	(3)	Paid Distribution Outside the Mails Including Sales Through Dealers and Carriers, Street Vendors, Counter Sales, and Other Paid Distribution Outside USPS®	992	985
	(4)	Paid Distribution by Other Classes Mailed Through the USPS (e.g. First-Class Mail®)		
c. Total Paid Distribution (*Sum of 15b (1), (2), (3), and (4)*)			2270	2131
d. Free or Nominal Rate Distribution (By Mail and Outside the Mail)	(1)	Free or Nominal Rate Outside-County Copies Included on PS Form 3541	105	95
	(2)	Free or Nominal Rate In-County Copies Included on PS Form 3541		
	(3)	Free or Nominal Rate Copies Mailed at Other Classes Through the USPS (e.g. First-Class Mail)		
	(4)	Free or Nominal Rate Distribution Outside the Mail (Carriers or other means)		
e. Total Free or Nominal Rate Distribution (Sum of 15d (1), (2), (3) and (4)			105	95
f. Total Distribution (Sum of 15c and 15e)			2375	2226
g. Copies not Distributed (See instructions to publishers #4 (page #3))			962	542
h. Total (Sum of 15f and g)			3337	2768
i. Percent Paid (15c divided by 15f times 100)			95.58%	95.73%

16. Publication of Statement of Ownership
    If the publication is a general publication, publication of this statement is required. Will be printed in the **October 2011** issue of this publication.
    ☐ Publication not required
17. Signature and Title of Editor, Publisher, Business Manager, or Owner
    Stephen R. Bushing
    Stephen R. Bushing –Inventory/Distribution Coordinator
    Date: September 16, 2011

I certify that all information furnished on this form is true and complete. I understand that anyone who furnishes false or misleading information on this form or who omits material or information requested on the form may be subject to criminal sanctions (including fines and imprisonment) and/or civil sanctions (including civil penalties).

PS Form 3526, September 2007 (Page 2 of 3)

Moving?

Make sure your subscription moves with you!

To notify us of your new address, find your **Clinics Account Number** (located on your mailing label above your name), and contact customer service at:

Email: journalscustomerservice-usa@elsevier.com

800-654-2452 (subscribers in the U.S. & Canada)
314-447-8871 (subscribers outside of the U.S. & Canada)

Fax number: 314-447-8029

Elsevier Health Sciences Division
Subscription Customer Service
3251 Riverport Lane
Maryland Heights, MO 63043

*To ensure uninterrupted delivery of your subscription, please notify us at least 4 weeks in advance of move.

ELSEVIER

Printed and bound by CPI Group (UK) Ltd, Croydon, CR0 4YY

03/10/2024

01040454-0014